Stammering in Young Children

A practical self-help programme for parents

by

Ann Irwin

D1392454

THORSONS PUBLISHING GROUP

First published 1988

© Ann Irwin 1988

British Library Cataloguing in Publication Data

Irwin, Ann
Stammering in young children.
1. Children. Stuttering. Therapy
I. Title
618.92′855406

ISBN 0-7225-1640-1

Published by Thorsons Publishing Limited, Wellingborough,
Northamptonshire NN8 2RQ, England

Printed in Great Britain by
Biddles Limited, Guildford, Surrey

3 5 7 9 10 8 6 4 2

Stammering in Young Chil

A practical self-hel

Dedication

To all the parents who overcome their children's stammers.

Sweet Benjamin, since thou art young,
And hast not yet the use of tongue,
Make it thy slave, whilst thou art free;
Imprison it, lest it do thee

John Hoskins

Contents

Foreword

This is a book for the parents of young children who fear that they may be beginning to stammer. It is written by a speech therapist who has devoted most of her long working life to helping those who are afflicted with this profoundly disturbing block to communication.

She is already the author of a book about a treatment she devised and perfected for adult stammerers. In this new book she describes a deceptively simple way to help young children, which could prevent them from becoming stammerers. Her Preventive Therapy is a method which could go a long way towards virtually eliminating developmental stammering in children and so, eventually, this prime cause of stammering in adults.

Ann Irwin, herself a mother of three children, has devised this programme from her observations that some parents, teachers and friends sometimes unwittingly foster early stammering in children by the stresses of drawing attention to their speech. But Preventive Therapy is more than just advice to remove these stresses. It is a carefully worked out system, elaborating six preventive techniques concerned with speech and others concerned with general behaviour, each fully illustrated with examples and supported by evidence from Mrs Irwin's own clinical experience.

The techniques are clearly explained, but removing pressures on children is not an easy matter, and most parents using these techniques will welcome the expert guidance of a speech therapist in reassuring them that they are using the techniques appropriately and at the right time. They should

be able to obtain this help by contacting their District
Speech Therapist through their local Health Authority.

Mrs Irwin's book is essential reading for parents who
recognize the signs of early stammering in their pre-school
children. The application of Preventive Therapy could spare
many people the distress of becoming confirmed stammerers
in later life.

Ruth Lesser, PhD, BA, BSc, MCST, ABPsS,
Head of Department of Speech,
The University of Newcastle upon Tyne

Introduction

People often ask me what is the cause of stammering and the answer is I do not know. Nobody knows. It remains a medical enigma despite 60 years of research, mostly in the USA. Stammering does seem to run in families and although this is not always the case, it happens often enough to make one feel certain that there must be an inherited tendency to stammer. Sometimes several members of one family stammer but, more often than not there are just one, two or three across an extended family and these are much more likely to be male than female. It could be the child's father or mother or, indeed, any relation but there is a tendency for the other relations who stammer to be 'sideways', as it were, to the child's immediate family, for example an uncle, a great uncle or a cousin.

It is believed that about one per cent of the adult population stammer and it has been estimated that it occurs in about four per cent of young children, so our first sign of reassurance is that three out of four children outgrow stammering spontaneously without help. But what of the one per cent who will not outgrow it without help? And what is this help?

I hope that Preventive Therapy, as set out in this book, will give a substantial part of the answer. Preventive Therapy is based on the conviction that the outcome of a stammer in a pre-school child depends not on the child himself but on the behaviour of the people around him, particularly his parents; that the stammer continues and increases while *pressures* are put on the child's speech; that the stammer decreases and continues to decrease when these pressures are removed. There is no doubt at all that if all the people around the pre-school child do all the right things then it is extremely likely that the child will outgrow the stammer.

The most vital speech therapy for stammering must surely be for young children because the onset of the problem occurs most frequently in the very young and it responds most readily to therapy during its early stages. Stammering begins from about two years onwards up to the age of nine. Any exceptions are rare. Most often the stammer begins between the ages of three and five.

Generally speaking, adults who stammer can learn to overcome and control the problem quite well but rarely outgrow it completely. Children over seven years and teenagers frequently outgrow stammering entirely but many do not. I find that the five to seven year age group respond excellently to Preventive Therapy and have almost as high a success rate as the under-fives. This may be because the stammer is less firmly established in these earlier years and possibly because educationally, and at home, less is expected of children at that age. The under-fives have every chance of outgrowing stammering completely.

People with established stammers may find it difficult to treat themselves successfully following a therapeutic programme from a book, but where a young child is concerned, when overcoming the stammer depends so much on the parents, a written programme of therapy should present few problems. It is only a matter of the parents reading and understanding the therapy and then putting it into practice.

Parents just do not know what to do about stammering but they are desperately keen to find out. First, they usually go to their doctor who frequently tries to reassure them by telling them that their child 'will grow out of it' and 'not to worry'. However, the weeks and the months pass and, for some, the child does not only *not* outgrow it but the stammer becomes more severe. The parents wait anxiously for the stammer to begin to improve and feel helpless because they do not know what to do.

It is the aim of Preventive Therapy to eliminate the stammer, before it develops and becomes established, by removing all the possible pressures on the child's speech. These are removed by or via the parents and will be discussed one by one. These pressures are not the *cause* of the stammer but, once a stammer exists, pressures on speech keep the stammer going and this is the reason that it is so important to know what they are and how to eliminate them. Parents are *in no way to blame* for these pressures; they do not even know that they exist and have no idea at all of what they are. The removal of the pressures creates the conditions that give the child the optimum chance of outgrowing the stammer.

Many speech therapists have long held the view that direct speech therapy is inappropriate for the very young child who stammers. Years ago, when I saw both the parents and the child, I found that my time spent with the *parents* was much more productive than my time spent with the *child*. As we talked together and discussed some of the things that helped or hindered their child's speech, it became more and more apparent that what made the stammer more marked was usually pressures put on the child's speech and that it was usually the parents who, unknowingly, created them.

The pressures we talked about were similar to those that had for many a year been discussed in the literature about stammering. It was sometimes said that we must not ask too much of the parents but, in practice, attempts to *lessen* the pressures were often insufficient to have a marked effect on the child's stammer. However, when we began with the parents to systematically and wholeheartedly *remove* the pressures, one by one, it made all the difference. Also we found that half doing the job was not enough; it appeared that full commitment to the cause was necessary. Then, with child after child completely overcoming his or her stammer, 'Preventive Therapy' seemed to be the appropriate phrase to describe what was happening. I believe that this success is directly attributable to clearly defining six speech pressures and to removing these pressures systematically, one at a time. This gives parents time to appreciate how important they are, and to work thoroughly on removing them.

We found that it was not even necessary for the child to attend the clinic but, instead, the parents came because it is they who carry out all the therapy. As a rule I see the child on one occasion only when the parents first visit me. This is because I want to meet the child and listen to his speech and to know who we are talking about in future meetings with his parents. If I see the child again, it is usually on the day he is discharged. The parents that I meet are, of course, those who have actively sought help. They are remarkable. They are very keen to do everything they can and, once they know what to do, they work very conscientiously at removing the speech pressures and, I don't want to disillusion you, it *is* hard work. It takes time and it takes concentration. Often both parents come to the clinic, but more often it is just the mother and it is she who takes the responsibility of telling the father all that we have talked about and it is she, again, who ensures that all the people in the child's environment are also taking off the pressures.

Preventive Therapy, particularly at first, may not always be readily accepted until it is understood. One happy father, on the day we discharged his six-year-old son, six months after he had totally lost his stammer, said, 'We never thought the day would come when James would be discharged, completely cured. To tell you the truth, now that his stammer has gone, I can tell you what we thought when we first met you. We just didn't believe what you said. When you asked us to stop telling him to slow down we were horrified. You were asking us to stop doing the *one* thing that stopped him stammering; we could not believe that you were asking that of us; it didn't make sense. We didn't know *what* to do after that and we talked about it for ages. We were so sure you were wrong but finally we decided to do what you had asked because there was no other advice to be had. So, if at any time *other* parents don't believe you, tell them to ring us and we will tell them to do what you say even if it seems to be the wrong advice!'

It is a great joy to parents and to myself to discharge a child knowing that the stammer has completely disappeared and has remained so over a period of months. When the child has been stammer-free, this is, totally free, for a period of six to nine months, the chances of it returning are virtually nil. I have only known it to return under extreme conditions, such as during World War II, when a few prisoners in Japanese prisoner of war camps began to stammer again even though they had lost their stammers in childhood. However, for practical purposes you could say that once a stammer has disappeared for nine months it has disappeared for good.

The alternative to losing a stammer is to have a problem throughout life. The size of the problem in adults varies according to the severity of the stammer and the personality of the subject. Some people who stammer take it more or less in their stride but others, who find their way to a speech therapy department, find it a source of constant embarrassment to say the least. To give just a few examples, a social worker I knew could not sleep at night because he was to speak in a court of law and feared that he would not be able to speak at the crucial moment; a medical consultant felt panic at the thought of having to lecture to medical students; a postman was happy to deliver letters as he was not required to speak, but feared to deliver parcels because he would have to ring the doorbell and speak to whoever answered. Anticipation and anxiety cause the biggest problems. An instance of this is of the man who sold his house and moved to a new street because he was unable to say his address; within months he was unable to say his new address.

Such situations need not arise if you take advantage of Preventive Therapy. I shall, throughout, call the child with a stammer 'Benjamin', after the inspiring poem at the beginning of this book, in preference to frequently repeating the phrase 'the child who has a stammer'. The word 'stammerer' I think should be avoided altogether on the grounds that we should refrain from labelling people. Once we have labelled them we tend to regard them in terms of the label we have given them. Thus, parents who think of their child as 'a stammerer' or refer to him or her as 'a stammerer' will tend to regard the child as abnormal instead of regarding him or her as a normal child who happens to have a stammer.

CHAPTER 1

The diagnosis of stammering

What is 'normal' speech?

Diagnosing stammering is not always as simple as people might think. Everyone is what speech therapists call 'normally non-fluent' and, on the whole, children are more non-fluent than adults. To explain what I mean, take the following example. A speech therapist friend of mine and I used to attend the same church and we had a minister who we thought of as a very fluent speaker. He was never at a loss for words, he did not seem to hesitate and his sermons usually lasted about 20 minutes. One day, when my friend and I had been discussing normal non-fluencies, she said that she was going to church the next Sunday and, instead of listening to the sermon, she was going to count the non-fluencies. She counted 52. If the minister was maintaining the average speed of 140 words per minute and he spoke for 20 minutes, then he was non-fluent for one of every 54 of his words. If a professional speaker, using notes and generally regarded as fluent can be this non-fluent, imagine the score for you or me, let alone our children. We are non-fluent in different ways. Some people say 'um' and 'er' between words; most of us 'um' and 'er' to some extent and also repeat sounds (wwwhen), repeat syllables (when when) and repeat phrases (when I was when I was). Most of us are aware that it is normal to be less than 100 per cent fluent but we have no idea at all just how non-fluent we generally are.

On occasion I have heard speakers, particularly politicians, on radio or television, repeating a phrase up to ten times. It is common, if you listen, to hear them repeating phrases up to five or six times. If you stop listening to the content of a conversation or speech and listen instead to the non-fluencies, you will be amazed at how many you will find. It is easiest to listen to people on radio and television as you can then devote your whole attention to the way that people are speaking rather than having to respond to what they are saying. Beware, however, of people who are not speaking spontaneously. You will not hear non-fluencies from a newsreader or someone who has learned or rehearsed what he is going to say. I remember listening to Sir Ralph Richardson, on the radio, and my attention was caught because I thought the speaker was controlling a stammer extremely well – all I could detect were very tiny blocks in the speech. I did not know who the speaker was until the end of the programme. If Sir Ralph was normally non-fluent to such an extent, imagine how non-fluent we must be!

If a politician can repeat a phrase ten times and not be regarded as having a stammer, how is it that Benjamin may repeat a phrase only three times and yet be regarded as stammering? If, as so often happens, there is stammering in the family, is the parent listening to normal speech and diagnosing it as stammering speech? Imagine a father who has a stammer; his son Benjamin repeats what he is saying, 'Mummy, mummy, mummy, I want to play to play to play with the ba ba ball.' The father, understandably fearful that his son is going to develop the same problem he has, begins to wonder, then to worry, then to diagnose. This diagnosis could be the beginning of a speech problem because once the child is labelled as having a stammer people begin to react to the child's speech, drawing attention to it and 'correcting' it. To take another example, imagine a family where the child repeats his words in exactly the same way that Benjamin did. But in this family nobody notices it, or, if they do notice, they regard it as normal because the child, after all, is very young and thus is expected to talk with non-fluencies. In each case the child's speech is exactly the same, yet in one family he is thought of as having a stammer, in another family he is thought of as having normal speech for a young child.

If you put ten people in a room together, play them a recording of speech and ask them to count the non-fluencies, you will most likely end up with ten different numbers. If you play them a recording of someone stammering and ask them to count the stammers, you will almost certainly end up with ten different numbers. I am sure that you will now understand that much depends on the listener – not just on the speaker – regarding the way we judge others' speech.

We must also bear in mind that we are not born with language ready made in our heads. A child learns language from the people around him, usually speaking words when he is about one year old, gradually progressing to phrases and then to complete sentences. He is not going to do this without a good deal of stumbling over words, searching for words, using the wrong words and, it must be stressed, hesitating over words. Many adults, when trying to speak a new language, would spend most of their time saying 'um' and 'er'. Without doubt it is possible for a child who does not have a stammer to be diagnosed as having one. Nevertheless, it is also true that many children who stammer have been regarded as normal speakers for a year or more before the stammer begins, so there must be something different happening to their speech pattern.

Things that can start a child stammering

Why is it that Benjamin develops a stammer when his brothers and sisters may not? Anything it seems can trigger it off. Parents, when asked what they think started it, say things like it started when he copied the speech of the boy next door; when a cat frightened him; when his granny died; when he was nearly run over by a car; when a dog bit him; when he got whooping cough; when his mother went into hospital; when the chip pan caught fire. Sometimes it is, 'When he started school' and sometimes it is simply, 'We just don't know.' From these examples we at least have some idea of the conditions under which stammering is sometimes said to begin, but exactly *why* it begins is still a mystery.

The symptoms

The stammer may develop gradually or it may come very suddenly. One mother said, 'I hardly noticed it to begin with;

I thought it was just normal speech. Then he started doing it more and it was months before we really thought he was stammering', but another mother said, 'His speech was fine until one day he just started stammering. It was so sudden that I wrote it down in my diary.' Further confusion commonly arises because often the stammer comes and goes: one minute the child is talking fluently and the next minute he is stammering. Periods of fluency vary in duration and may last for minutes, hours, weeks or even months. Parents are often excellent witnesses. They know if the stammer occurs at the beginning of words, at the beginning of sentences, in-between words, approximately how frequently it occurs and what tends to cause it, such as excitement. They also recognize what type of stammer it is when they listen to different forms of stammering. However, parents can only rarely describe in their own words what the stammer symptoms are. The most usual stammer symptoms in children are:

- repetition of sounds (m m m mummy)
- repetition of syllables (mum mum mum mummy) and single syllable words (why why why)
- repetition of words (only only only)
- repetition of phrases (I want I want I want)
- prolongation of consonant sounds (m ummy)
- prolongation of vowel sounds (mu mmy)
- inappropriate pauses.

A child may have one of these symptoms or a mixture of several of them. In addition, he may cover his mouth with his hand as if he is ashamed of his speech and, rarely, he may hold his throat as if he is trying to help the words to get out.

In true stammering there is virtually always *some* tension when these symptoms are produced. The degree of tension will vary from child to child and will range from quite slight to quite severe. If there is no tension at all, the child may not be stammering but just be somewhat more non-fluent than the average child. It is not always possible to recognize the difference between stammering and normal non-fluencies. Strangely, repetitions of whole words of more than one syllable are often not recognized as being stammered words. A child calling, 'Mummy mummy mummy come here' would give the listener the impression of excitement or panic but would not sound like stammering.

A much more positive symptom of stammering than either repetitions or prolongations is blocking. Blocks occur at points where, in normal speech, two speech organs meet together gently, but in stammering instead of meeting gently they come together with tension. This may happen when the two lips meet as for 'p' and 'b', when the tip of the tongue is raised against the hard palate as for 't' and 'd', and when the back of the tongue is raised against the soft palate as for 'k' and 'g'. Blocks occur particularly at the level of the vocal cords in the larynx (in the throat, commonly called the Adam's apple), where in normal speech they vibrate to produce the voice. These blocks may be silent or they may be voiced. They are frequently apparent in older children and adults who stammer but they do sometimes occur in young children and, when severe, sometimes veins on the sides of the neck stand out and/or the eyes bulge. Once the troublesome word is out, all the tension disappears and the speech muscles return to normal.

Stammering can happen with any word, in any part of a sentence, but it tends to occur most at the beginnings of speech. It is usually more frequent at the beginning of a sentence and it almost always occurs at the beginning of a word, either on the first sound or on the first vowel. When stammering occurs before or between words, but not on the word itself, it usually takes the form of a repeated or prolonged vowel sound, for example a a a a or a .

There is no cause to be more concerned about a severe stammer than about a mild stammer – both respond to Preventive Therapy.

PREVENTIVE THERAPY PART ONE
The pressures on speech

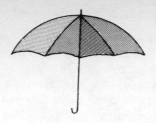

CHAPTER 2

The Umbrella

The Preventive Therapy of:
- learning to stop reacting negatively to the stammer
- learning to identify what makes the stammer increase and what makes the stammer decrease

What the Umbrella symbol stands for

An umbrella keeps off the rain, the snow, the hail and the wind: it protects us from the elements. Preventive Therapy keeps off the harmful reactions of other people; it protects the child who stammers from people trying to make him 'stop doing it', and so I feel the Umbrella is a very appropriate image. The stammering child needs protection from every pressure upon his speech because these pressures make him feel anxious about speaking and so only help make the stammer worse.

I think of the Umbrella as the *overall* protection for the child of *not reacting negatively to the stammer* and I think of the child coming under the protection of that Umbrella, being protected from the *specific* pressures on his speech.

Learning to stop reacting negatively to the stammer

What do I mean by learning to stop reacting negatively to the stammer? Well, let's take a look at Benjamin's speech from his own point of view and then from the point of view of the people around him, particularly that of his parents.

Picture then, Benjamin. We'll say he is four years old and lives with his brother John, who is six, and his mother and father. It is a happy household and the family have lots of good times together. John goes to school and father goes to work, so Benjamin and his mother have a lot of time on their own. Sometimes friends and relations call at the house to spend time with them and, at other times, Benjamin and his Mum go out together shopping or to the park to play or sometimes to the swimming pool where Benjamin's mother is teaching him to swim. Life is good. It's fun. Benjamin, as he is only four, takes each day as it comes, he doesn't think too much about yesterday, or too much about tomorrow, unless something exciting is happening. He is going to start nursery school next term and he is quite excited about that but doesn't give it too much thought.

His heart beats and his lungs breathe; his eyes see and his ears hear but he has never thought about any of these things. He is much too young to know anything about his heart and lungs and eyes and ears. He talks too. Of course he has never paid any attention to talking; he is much too young. Talking just happens, it is not something you have to think about. If Benjamin thought about seeing he would be glad that he could see; if he thought about hearing he would be glad that he could hear; if he thought about talking he would be glad that he could speak, for speech is the gateway to self expression and the development of relationships, but Benjamin knows nothing about such things. Neither does he know that some of the words he utters take longer to say than other words, that sometimes he repeats sounds and prolongs vowels. These have never even crossed his mind, he has never noticed them. But his parents have noticed them.

Benjamin's parents used to be a bit concerned about his speech but now they are much more concerned because the hesitations haven't stopped as they had hoped. John didn't talk like that when he was four, he never had anything wrong with his speech. And, it is a funny thing, but John has never noticed the way Benjamin speaks; or, if he has noticed, he has never said anything. Yet the friends and relations who call at the house have noticed it, they have often said, 'Have you noticed the way Benjamin talks?', and recently they've been saying, 'I should stop him doing that, if I were you, before it gets worse.'

Benjamin's parents would prefer not to be told what to do about it, but nevertheless, they had been thinking on the same lines. They hope he'll grow out of it but they do know of adults who never grew out of it and they would hate that to happen to Benjamin. They begin to think about what it will be like if Benjamin continues to stammer. Will he get teased at nursery school? When he gets to school will the stammer hold him back? When he gets older will it make him shy with girls? Will it stop him from getting a job? Of course, he may grow out of it, the doctor said he would, they think, but wouldn't it be awful if he didn't? So Benjamin's parents wonder what they should do. The only thing left, it seems to them, is to try to help by telling Benjamin what he should and shouldn't do. They tell him to slow down, to take his time, to say it again, to relax, to stop being silly. They are often rewarded by magic moments when Benjamin repeats the words he has been stammering on without any stammering. Naturally they think they are on the right tracks and this 'helpful correction' becomes a part of family life.

How, though, do children themselves *feel* about 'helpful correction'? Imagine Benjamin running to his mummy and saying, 'M m mummy m m my ball has gone. J J Johnny has thrown it over over the garden wa wa wa wall', and she replies, 'Take your time, Benjamin, say it again slowly.' Here is Benjamin, desperate to communicate, set only on mummy coming to the rescue and fetching his ball back. But his message falls on deaf ears. It is his stammer, not his message, that gets the response. How frustrating it must be for him.

Imagine his mother's car is damaged by somebody reversing into it. She is both angry and upset and longing to share her emotions with someone. Luckily, when she gets home her husband is in. She rushes up to him and says, 'Darling, I'm furious; some idiot has just reversed into the car and done quite a bit of damage.' Her husband listens, then replies, 'Darling, do slow down, you are talking much too quickly.' Unlikely? Frustrating? Infuriating? Yes of course, but that is what happens to Benjamin a great deal of the time. Little wonder that he learns to feel badly about talking. If this kind of response was typical of her husband's responses, you can just imagine that eventually she would feel, 'What is the good of trying?' and get more and more tense, anticipating the unwanted and unacceptable response from her husband. Her jaw would tighten and her hands would screw up at the thought of what is coming – and she hasn't even got a stammer; imagine what it must be like for Benjamin when the words will not come out properly on top of this. The listener has not responded appropriately to what has been said. Communication, as it should be, has been thrown away.

Correcting Benjamin's speech

In the clinic where I work, I think the hardest thing for parents to accept, in the early stages of therapy, is that all 'correction' has to stop. They think I am asking them to give up the one thing that actually stops, or frequently stops, the stammer. It often takes time for them to come to terms with this new idea, but, I have to explain, 'correction' is only the short-term benefit. If it was helping overall the stammer would be improving, but they have come to the clinic because the stammer is worsening so it is the long-term benefit that we have to be concerned with.

When parents begin to 'correct' Benjamin for stammering, he does not even know that there is anything wrong with his speech. Even if he is a particularly sensitive child who has noticed his non-fluencies, he would have no cause for concern. His speech is fine as far as he is concerned, but he keeps getting 'corrected' for something he has done; what he has done may be a mystery to him but, as the 'correction' continues, he gradually becomes aware of what it is that he is doing and of which his parents disapprove. He thus begins to try not to do it and, in the effort of trying, the tension increases, stress about speaking develops and the stammer symptoms increase in frequency and severity. The more he stammers the more he gets 'corrected' and, the more he gets 'corrected' the more he stammers. In this vicious circle Benjamin becomes much more aware of the stammer and begins to feel badly about speaking. So the short-term benefit of 'correcting' and being rewarded with a fluent word is an extremely high price to pay for the long-term future of both speech stress and increased stammer. This is why in

Preventive Therapy I say *stop all correction of the stammer*.

It is not only Benjamin's parents who need to stop 'correcting' – *everyone*, that is everyone without exception, should stop. Aunts, uncles, grannies, grandfathers, friends, neighbours and acquaintances, if they take any notice at all of the stammer, should be requested not to do so, and an explanation be given if necessary. Usually people, once they understand, will immediately stop. If anyone is in the habit of 'correcting' frequently, then it may take them a week or two to remember to stop. Sometimes relations will argue the point, insisting that it helps; if this happens, you need to explain. If they will not accept the explanation it has always, in my experience, been enough to say, 'That is what the speech therapist told us, and that is what we are determined to do.'

Sometimes other *children* notice the stammer and begin reacting negatively to it, although children under seven rarely notice it at all. Older children rarely 'correct' it but are more likely to tease or mimic. My first instinct is to enlist their help: 'Look Bobby, you know, don't you, that Benjy has a little bit of trouble getting his words out at times, well, we've been told that he will grow out of it if nobody takes any notice of it. It would be a great help if you would stop teasing him about it, would you do that? Thanks for your help.' Asking other children for their help often works wonderfully well. If it doesn't, I would temporarily stop Benjamin from playing with the children who tease him and, if possible, substitute these older friends with children nearer to Benjamin's age. I would certainly try to find a way of protecting Benjamin from children who insist on drawing his attention to his speech and who make him feel badly about it.

The great advantage of Preventive Therapy for pre-school children is that every single person in the child's environment can be controlled. All can be stopped from 'correcting' the stammer. This is sometimes all that is required. The 'correction' stops and the stammer decreases and goes on decreasing. Once the child is at nursery school the outlook is probably as good. If the child is already at, or soon to start, nursery school, this is easily dealt with. The teachers are few in number and you only have to ask them not to 'correct' the stammer, nor react to it in any way and do their best to avoid anything that makes the stammer increase. Once the child is at 'big' school the situation is different. What I say in this book applies as much to the child in his first few years of school as to the pre-school child, but the difference is that the environment can no longer be so completely controlled. No matter what precautions are taken, and they should be taken, one cannot ensure that the teachers and the children will not react against the stammer.

Although both parents share the responsibility for all that is required in Preventive Therapy, it is usually the mother's lot to contact people, to explain about not 'correcting', and to ensure that they do as requested. In addition it is usually the mother who is at home with Benjamin and who has to watch her own behaviour towards him all the time. It is very hard work, needing constant vigilance, and I can only admire the way that mothers set to work with determination and vigour for the sake of their children.

If the father is unemployed or self-employed he can then work as hard as the mother on Benjamin's speech, but in most cases he is out at work and can only help for a few hours in the evenings. Fathers too, on the whole, are able to put their worries aside. They are practical enough to feel that everything possible is being done so there is no point in worrying about it. Mothers tend to be much more emotional and anxious and are less able to put their worries aside, but these worries decrease as the stammer improves.

Two case histories

Here are two case histories showing how stammering improved when people stopped reacting to it, which support what I have been saying.*

Susan

Susan was five years old and stammered a great deal of the time. When she stammered she repeated the first sound of a word quickly and several times. Her mother and I discussed in detail the need for everyone to stop reacting to the stammer or taking any notice of it. Theirs was a very big family and they met frequently so Susan's mother had to tell more than twenty relations, as well as many friends, about the therapy. I

*In the case histories the child's name has been changed. Also, minor details have sometimes been changed in order to avoid identification but these do not alter the substance of these true stories.

contacted Susan's teacher, who, in fact, was not reacting to the stammer. Susan continued to stammer and I was rather surprised that there was no improvement because I knew that, before therapy started, a lot of relations and friends had been 'correcting' the stammer and making comments about it. Then one day Susan's mother came in to the clinic and said, 'I've discovered that two of Susan's aunts are still taking notice of the stammer. They have not been "correcting" it but they think it sounds very attractive and they have been laughing when she does it and asking her to do it again. I have told them they have got to stop.' They stopped. A week later Susan's mother said the stammer was already improving; she was stammering less often. Two weeks after that Susan was hardly stammering at all and four weeks later there was no sign of stammer, it had stopped. A check some months later revealed that the stammer had not returned.

David

David was not quite five. On their first visit to the clinic I noted that David's stammer was particularly severe for such a young child. He was getting blocks at vocal cord level, in the larynx, his speech sounded very tense and 'strangled' and he was having to force the words through his throat.

He lived with one older sister, one older brother and two parents and they all 'corrected' him. His mother was so concerned about the stammer and so desperate for him to stop that she not only 'corrected' him but also got very cross with him for stammering. She didn't really *feel* cross but she thought that if she sounded cross he would be more likely to stop stammering. For good measure she told him that he was silly to speak like that. He tried 'terribly hard not to do it'; I know, because that is what he actually said to me!

His mother was so loving and caring and she had been doing everything she could possibly think of to stop the stammer but, like so many other parents, she did the wrong things. Two weeks later she returned and said, 'It is just amazing; we all stopped taking any notice of David's speech and for ten days he didn't stammer at all. Then at the weekend he went to a party and got rather excited and he has been stammering a bit since then, but not very much.'

There is no magic. It will no doubt take months, or even a

year or more, for David to completely overcome the stammer but it is an excellent start. His mother is surprised and delighted and wishes they had known, from the start, that stammering should not be 'corrected'. Nevertheless parents should not feel guilty about 'correcting' – they 'correct' because it seems the only thing to do and they are doing their very best to help. The two examples of what happened to Susan and David are a little exceptional because the improvement was so sudden, but they do serve to show what *can* happen when children are made aware of their speech, and how changes can come about when they are no longer made aware of it.

Less obvious ways of 'correcting'

Not 'correcting' the stammer is only a part of the wider picture of *not reacting negatively to the stammer*. These days people talk a great deal about 'body language', and it is a fact that we frequently communicate our feelings and thoughts by our bodily movements or posture. A child who is hopping along the street on one foot and giggling doesn't have to say, 'I'm feeling happy', we can see that for ourselves. When a mother looks at her newborn baby we know she is thinking he is the most beautiful baby in the world without her saying a word. A man parks his car, goes to the parking meter, puts his hands in his pockets, looks around, and we know he has no change to put in the meter even though he has not said a thing.

Sometimes we use body language deliberately. For example, when we cup a hand around our ear it means, 'I cannot hear you'; when we beckon with a finger it means, 'Come here', but for the most part we use body language unknowingly and other people can often tell, for example, if we are tense or relaxed, if we are nervous and, to some extent, how we are feeling and what we are thinking. We can also often read facial expressions. Love, for instance, is not likely to be confused with hate and joy, anger, resignation, disappointment, fear and expectation all show.

How does our body language relate to *not reacting negatively to the stammer*? Let me give some examples. Parents sometimes say to me, 'I know it's awful but I just cannot stand staying in the room when Benjamin is stammering.

I stay as long as I can and then I just have to walk out, I cannot bear to see him like that.' When people do not actually leave the room they sometimes want to get out at the first possible opportunity because Benjamin is there stammering and he takes what seems like minutes to get out just a few words. If the listener is too polite to just walk out, she* stands in the doorway, one hand on the door, all ready to make a quick getaway just as soon as Benjamin has said what he was trying to say.

One mother said to me, 'I *never* react to his stammer, I go and look out of the window and wait until he has finished speaking.' This is a perfect example of body language. She was saying to him, in effect, 'I do not want to watch you speaking so I'll just stand patiently with my back to you until you have finished.' It had not even crossed her mind that in a normal conversation we watch the speaker, not turn our back on him. She thought that she was not reacting to the stammer.

Benjamin is blocking a great deal; the words are really stuck. His mother is so upset, she feels so sorry for him. She is watching Benjamin as he struggles. As she watches and listens a tear comes into her eye and she brushes it away. Body language.

Other parents look frustrated, anxious, annoyed. Their facial expressions convey to Benjamin how he is being regarded. More subtle body language, but no more acceptable, is to sigh with relief when his fluency returns. In all of these examples Benjamin must slowly but surely begin to realize that his speech brings unusual responses from those around him; these responses make him aware that his speech is unacceptable. Preventive Therapy insists that they should be avoided so far as is possible.

How the child who stammers feels

What is it like for Benjamin when he feels badly about his speech? We have to look no further than how *we* might feel in

---

*Throughout, 'she' is used in preference to 'he or she' because it is usually the mother who spends most time with the child, but what is said could equally apply to the father, relative or male friend of the family.

similar cirumstances when speaking situations make us apprehensive. Most of us know what it is like to feel nervous about speaking. Perhaps we have to speak in public or give a lecture and some of us are all but terrified. We wonder if we are going to make fools of ourselves, if our mouths will go dry just at the crucial moments, if we will be able to remember what we intend to say. If a public speaker is nervous and unsure of himself he is almost certain to speak non-fluently and someone in the audience is sure to make the remark, 'He was so nervous he was stammering.' A case of mistaken diagnosis! Even quite ordinary speaking situations, such as a dinner party, make some people feel uncomfortable as they anticipate the pressure of having to speak, preferably with sparkle, to people they do not know. We worry about our speech when much is expected of us and so does Benjamin. We all need to enjoy speaking and to feel relaxed about it; it makes all the difference to our confidence. And if Benjamin needs anything he needs to feel confident about speaking.

While we need to protect children against feeling badly about their speech, it must be said that they have varying degrees of awareness of their stammers. Some appear to have no awareness of it at all and it is important, if possible, to keep it that way, while others are so aware of stammering that should their speech not be understood or should the word become very difficult to get out, will give up talking altogether saying, 'Never mind, it doesn't matter' or, 'I can't say it.'

Ignoring Benjamin's stammer

People sometimes advise parents to 'ignore the stammer'. This is good advice as far as it goes but it does not go nearly far enough. It means 'act as if it isn't there' and, although this is often an appropriate thing to do, it does not meet all the needs and it is negative advice. The positive alternative is to *accept* the stammer; there is, in any case, no choice unless, that is, to continue to fight and be distressed by it. Once the parents have accepted Benjamin's stammer, you need to observe it so that you can find ways of helping; then you should feel *free* to help. If a child stops speaking, because he feels unable to continue with speech, surely it is more reassuring to say, for example, 'Never mind, you can tell me later' or, 'Should I say that word for you?' or, 'Some words *are* difficult to say', than to pretend that the stammer does not exist or 'to ignore it'. If parents were ignoring this cry for help they would have to say something ridiculous like, 'Everything is fine, there is nothing wrong.' In this instance, of course, the child was aware of his stammer. It would be unwise to 'help out' with a child who is unaware of his stammer, and 'helping out' should be kept to an absolute minimum and only used if the child is distressed and if he gains relief from this kind of response.

If we can learn to treat the stammer as *normal speech*, and the more we treat it as normal the more normal it becomes, we are doing a great deal to help because the child, in feeling that his speech is acceptable to his parents, is relieved from speech stress. It is when we treat the stammer as *abnormal* that we court trouble.

The kinds of things that make it better, the kinds of things that make it worse

We are, then, beginning to see some of the behaviours that *make the stammer increase* and some that *make the stammer decrease* but it is also necessary for Benjamin's parents to identify, so far as is possible, what else seems to make it increase and decrease. Most people who stammer have 'good patches' and 'bad patches'; these may last from a few hours up to a few weeks or even months and often defy logic. There seems to be no definite reason at all why it happens. Nevertheless there are usually other factors at work that we are able to identify and these are very useful to know about because they provide us with guidelines to teach us which situations we should try to encourage and which situations we should try to avoid. It would be helpful to write down your own list so that, read daily, it will act as a reminder. Also, if you both write down the situations, you can discuss your lists together, when Benjamin is in bed and asleep, and decide what action you can take. Your list could read something like this:

Increase
- Whén tired
- When excited
- When he cannot watch a
  particular TV programme
- When he gets smacked
- Playing with other
  children outside
- When Aunty Mary
  comes

Decrease
- When he is playing alone
  with his cars
- When he plays with (his
  brother) John
- Saturdays
- When he is being read his
  bedtime story

In a family household we have got to be practical and there is no way Benjamin can, or should, always have his own way, but we can work towards making things easier for him so far as his speech is concerned. He should receive several benefits as a result of the implications of the above list.

Now suppose that Benjamin's parents, having made the list, are sitting down together to discuss whether it is possible to tackle it and, if so, what to do. Perhaps their ideas would run something like this:

Stammer increases:
When tired
Strategy:
- Try to avoid particularly late nights
- Avoid bedtime excitement, which tends to keep him awake
- Try coming home to lunch after nursery school so that he can relax *before* doing the shopping
- When tired after running: we cannot stop Benjamin's fun but we could try not to talk with him while he is out of breath

When excited
Strategy:
* If nobody *else* gets excited Benjamin's excitement will decrease; try this
* Play down rather than build up excitement over special events, for example outings, birthdays and parties. At Christmas start talking about what he wants a week or two before, not six weeks before the day

TV programmes
Strategy:
* There are arguments about this because John wants another channel. Explain to both boys that fair is fair and they can each choose their preferred programmes on alternate days

When he gets smacked
Strategy:
* Think of a way that smacking can be stopped and substituted with a punishment that does not increase the stammer – perhaps by withdrawing a privilege (for example, 'no sweets today'), along with an explanation that he has been naughty and had already been warned that he would go without his sweets if he didn't do as he had been asked

Playing outside
Strategy:
* If Benjamin is determined to play with other children outside we may increase the stammer further by refusing to let him go. If he is not too fussy about it we could try to cut it down or cut it out, suggesting something else he could do instead. We mustn't stop him mixing with people, perhaps we could try inviting just one or two children to tea

When Aunty Mary comes
Strategy:
* I wonder why Benjamin always stammers when Aunty Mary comes? Next time she visits I will stay with them all the time or listen to what they say to each other and try to discover what it may be. (One 'Aunty Mary' used to tease a little boy and keep him guessing as to whether or not she

had brought him a present; he used to start the conversation with, 'Ha ha ha ha ha ha have you brought brought brought me a me a present?')

Stammer decreases
When playing alone with his cars
Strategy:
- He sits on the floor, in a world of his own, talking to himself and making car noises and so on, all completely fluently, with no sign of stammer. Can we encourage that situation so that he is completely fluent more of the time? We could make sure that we do not interrupt him while he is playing and we could buy him a garage so that he may spend more time with his cars

When he plays just with John
Strategy:
- We do sometimes interrupt Benjamin and John when they are playing together so let's really try to stop doing that. We could occasionally buy them a game that is best for only two players to encourage them to play together more frequently

Saturdays
Strategy:
- What is different about Saturdays? He usually sleeps later. Then he spends a great deal of his time with his father, 'helping' to do the gardening, cleaning the car and usually some household repairs. Let's keep Saturday as it is

When he is being read his bedtime story
Strategy:
- He chats away at these times, talking about the stories and he has very little stammer then. We could easily give him a bit more time when we do this

Some of these suggestions may not be suitable in your case but they will help you to see how you can act positively. Study your own list and, in the light of this approach, decide what to do. You have to see what suits your own particular household and be guided by results, but do not expect quick results. We are looking for ways of decreasing the stammer, there is nothing that we can do to *stop* it in a short period of time.

Everything which decreases it is grist to the mill and is therefore worth working on, but it is best to carry out ideas in a relaxed and flexible way without upsetting the rest of the household unduly or completely exhausting yourselves.

Increase and decrease of stammer also depends, to some extent, on the *rate* at which the child speaks. Before they know better, almost all parents 'correct' the rate. Even when they do know better, the temptation to slow Benjamin down is great. 'If *only* he would slow down', they say, 'I'm sure he would be almost all right.' Asking him to speak slowly, apart from making him aware that you consider there is something wrong with his speech, is really asking the impossible. If you try to change the rate of your own speech you will discover how very difficult it is; try reducing your natural rate of speech by thirty per cent, and see how long you can keep it up! Five minutes? Ten minutes? Half an hour? A week? A year? People find it almost impossible to do for any length of time and yet this is what some people expect and hope Benjamin will do, and he is only four! Nevertheless, if you are a very quick speaker, you should do your very best to concentrate on your rate of speech and try to slow it down. It is unrealistic to hope that Benjamin will slow down if he lives in the same house as a rapid speaker.

It is certain that stammering becomes more pronounced when the rate of speech is increased. *Increase in rate usually occurs when the child is excited.* So is there anything you can do to slow down Benjamin's speech without actually telling him to slow down? The answer is 'yes' but it is a qualified 'yes'. You may expect some good to come out of it but you may not expect Benjamin to talk as slowly as you would wish.

Some strategies:
- You can try to curtail the excitement
- Keep calm and refrain from getting excited yourself
- Do not raise your voice
- Reduce the rate of your own speech, which is not difficult for a short period of time, and it gives him a good pattern to copy
- Do not make him hurry over anything: it is pointless to try to slow his speech if you are saying, 'Hurry up and get ready for bed' or, 'If we are quick there will be time for just one more game.' It is essential that you do not, at any

time, put pressure on him to speak more quickly, which tends to occur when parents are impatient. He must always feel that he has plenty of time to speak, both when he is fluent and when he is stammering

If Benjamin is quick and very active in everything he does, not just speech, you can try to slow down many of his activities, without singling out speech, and you could try this on a reward system. Let me give an example.

A case history

Polly

I know a little girl called Polly. She is six and she had quite a severe stammer, which has almost gone now. Her parents said that every single thing she did, she did quickly – she spoke quickly, ate quickly, never sat still on a chair but twisted either her legs, body, arms or hands. When she stood, she stood on one foot, swinging the other foot to and fro in the air. She ran *to* school, she ran *home* from school. She was never still – even in her sleep she moved about a lot. Both parents came to the clinic for our discussions on Preventive Therapy. They had already made sure that tartrazine had been eliminated from Polly's diet (the colour additive E102 reported to be a possible cause of hyperactivity in children).

We agreed that if we could somehow get Polly to slow her other activities down she might then begin to speak a little more slowly. So, we made a large picture of a cardboard clown and sent it to Polly by post, together with lots of cardboard discs valued at 5p and 10p. The clown was all ready for her to colour in and the cardboard discs were ready to stick on him, 5p for buttons and 10p for pompons. Polly's mother made a list of the activities she wanted slowed down and explained to Polly that she would get a 10p disc for every difficult task she managed and a 5p disc for the easier tasks. At the end of the week they would count how much money the Slow Down Clown had collected and give that amount of money to Polly. I'm afraid it got rather expensive!

Once Polly managed to achieve and maintain a particular task she would stop getting discs for it and a new task would be added to the list. After a few weeks Polly always *walked* to and from school, she did not even look like she wanted to run and *walking* was now the natural thing for her to do. In a similar way there were many more successes so that her other 'quick' activities were now under control and, along with the general slowing down came a considerable slowing down of speech, not a vast difference but sufficient for her parents to be aware of it.

Mothers go to a great deal of trouble and give a lot of thought to how best they can help their Benjamin. One mother I knew was worried because her four-year-old son was due to go on an outing to the beach with a large group of children. She knew that he would get very excited about it, that this would speed up his speech rate and make him stammer. She knew that the bigger the group the more excited he would get. So, she decided not to let him go on the outing; instead she arranged for her sister and her small son to join them and they went on an outing to the beach – just the four of them.

The importance of the Umbrella

I think that now you will realize just how important it is to use the Umbrella to protect your child from *general* pressures upon his speech that cause him stress. Parents find that these ideas are new to them and they like to go over the same points several times before their way of thinking changes and the suggestions become a way of life. It may therefore be helpful to read these chapters two or three times. Changing one's attitude takes time and nobody should worry if their goal takes some time to achieve or if mistakes are made along the way.

To summarize, the main objectives are:

- To learn to stop 'correcting' the stammer and make sure that nobody else 'corrects' it
- To try to avoid showing disapproval of, and anxiety about, the stammer through body language
- To take note of what makes the stammer *increase* and what makes it *decrease*, so that you have guidelines to help you
- To remember that working *indirectly* on speech rate is likely to be of some help

If you implement these suggestions, without doubt, you can

expect some improvement in the stammer. Sometimes these positive steps are all that is needed but, usually, it is also necessary to remove *specific* pressures and these are discussed in the next six chapters.

It is best to work on the Umbrella therapy until you feel that you have it quite well under control, but not necessarily to perfection, before moving on. It often takes two or three weeks to make these changes.

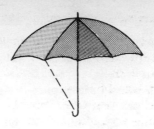

CHAPTER 3

Questions

Learning to reduce the number of questions you ask

Every time you ask Benjamin a question he has got to reply, so *asking questions* is a pressure on speech. Benjamin has not really got any option because he is expected to answer when you ask him something. We want him to talk, and to enjoy talking, but not be *made* to talk.

There is no doubt at all that asking questions increases stammering and for this reason they should be greatly reduced. I am not suggesting for a moment that questions should be stopped altogether – that would be unnatural. If Benjamin falls over you are going to say, 'Are you all right?' If he cries you are going to say, 'What's the matter?' Naturally we are certain to ask *some* questions but we should cut out the unnecessary questions, particularly by the parents as it is usually they who ask most of the questions.

We do not, however, want to cut out the amount of conversation that you and Benjamin are used to, and it is therefore necessary to learn how to replace the questions with conversation that is not put in question form. When Benjamin comes to the clinic, I never say, 'Hello Benjamin, how are you?', I say something like, 'Hello Benjamin, I'm glad you could come.' I do not say, 'Would you like to play with these toys?', I say, 'I've put some toys on the table, if you would like to play with them.' I do not ask, 'Would you like to sit on this little chair?', I say, 'Here is a little chair, just right for you', and so on. I am saying *as much* as I would if I were asking questions but I am *not* asking any questions and I am not putting any pressure on him to speak. Benjamin is free to talk if he feels so inclined but, importantly, he is free to remain quiet if he prefers. When I am explaining this aspect of Preventive Therapy to parents who come to the clinic, I try to demonstrate what I am getting at by saying something like, 'This is perhaps a little exaggerated, in order to get my point across, but this could be what a mother would say to her child when it is nearly time to go to nursery school.'

'Why aren't you ready for nursery?'
'Why aren't you dressed properly?'
'Where are your shoes?'
'Why have you got odd socks on?'
'What did you do that for?'
'Hurry up! Hurry up!'
'Have you got your apple?'
'Where did you put your book?'
'Why haven't you finished your breakfast?'
'Why don't you do as you're told?'

Then you meet Benjamin coming out of nursery, and what do mothers say?

'Have you had a nice day?'
'Did you eat your dinner?'
'What did you have for dinner?'
'What did you do today?'
'Was Mark at nursery today?'
'Have you forgotten anything to bring home?'
'Shall we go shopping?'
'Would you like some sweets?'

The point of this message is not lost on parents! It usually brings smiles and the response, 'That's me, that's just what I do! I never realized. I'd never thought about it before.' Parents do not realize the enormous number of questions they ask in the course of a day, and they can easily ask a hundred or more.

Let us now take a look at what a mother might have said to a child, before and after nursery school, *instead* of the above, and *without* asking questions.

'We are going to nursery soon; you should be getting ready.'

'You are not even dressed properly.'
'I don't know where you put your shoes.'
'Ben! You've got odd socks on!'
'I don't know what made you do that.'
'We had better not waste time, we will be late.'
'I've put your apple on the hall table.'
'And I've put your book with it.'
'I see you haven't finished your breakfast.'
'I wish you would do as you are told.'

Then, after nursery school:

'I've had a nice day; I hope you have.'
'I expect you ate up all your dinner after that small
    breakfast.'
'You probably had steak pie and potatoes for dinner; I just
    had a sandwich.'
'I'll bet you've been painting again today.'
'I haven't seen Mark today; I hope he is better again.'
'I see you are bringing home a new book.'
'I've got a little shopping to do so we will go to the shop before
    we go home.'
'You can have some sweets today if you like.'

Benjamin would no doubt prefer to have fewer comments
made to him both before and after nursery, even if they are
not questions. The suggested alternatives to questions are
included because mothers so frequently say that they do ask
a lot of questions both before and after school and they ask
what they could say instead. Mothers are very keen to show
an interest in what their children have been doing at school
and some are a little reluctant to stop saying, 'Have you had a
nice day?' If you really want to say that, do please say it. I am
not asking that you stop showing an interest or that you stop
asking questions altogether, just that you greatly reduce the
number of your questions. It often happens, however, that
when Benjamin *is* asked, 'Did you have a nice day?' he just
answers, 'It was all right' or 'OK' and does not give any
further information. Oftentimes, it seems, he prefers to
volunteer information rather than to be pressured into giving
it. He is, in any case, probably thinking about what to do next
rather than what he has already done.
  One mother said to me recently, 'Since I stopped asking
Jack a lot of questions he has started talking a lot more and

tells me all sorts of things about nursery school that he never told me before. The less I ask, the more he seems to talk. What is more, I have stopped asking his elder brother questions too. He doesn't have any problems with his speech but he used to answer my questions with one word or a shrug. Now that I don't ask him questions he tells me quite a lot. The difference it has made is really interesting, he talks so much more now.'

This example illustrates how parents gain insight as they proceed with Preventive Therapy, learning as they go along what helps and what hinders, and they sometimes tell me amusing stories about what they have thought up to avoid asking a question. One mother always asked Benjamin, after nursery school, what he had eaten for dinner. She was determined not to miss out this interest she always showed, but she couldn't think of a way of asking him about his dinner without asking a question. Finally, she went to the school at dinner time, walked round the back to where the kitchen was and peered through the window to see what the children were going to have to eat. Then she was able to say to Benjamin, 'I'll bet you had mince and mashed potatoes for dinner.' I never fail to wonder at the ingenuity of mothers!

Before you can have the insight and before the stammer benefits from therapy, there comes the hard work of learning how to cut down and rephrase questions and, of course, sustaining concentration while you are putting the therapy into practice. There is no doubt that it is hard work for about three or four weeks. People cannot think what to say instead of a question, then they find themselves asking questions and wish they hadn't and then, gradually, they manage to cut down on asking questions. Often they look for an immediate change in the stammer, which may, but probably will not, come so quickly. They worry too about other people asking questions. One mother told me that her family had returned from a holiday abroad when she took her little boy in to his nursery school just to say that he would be back the next day. The teacher showed a tremendous interest in what Benjamin had been doing for his holiday. The mother stood, almost rooted to the spot in horror, as the teacher asked him, 'Where did you go? Did you go abroad? Did you go in an aeroplane? Did you like it? Was the weather hot? Were you near the sea?' Feeling unsure about what to do, Benjamin's mother took his hand as quickly as possible to lead him away, saying to the teacher, 'We must be off now; I'll have to be careful what I say to him as the speech therapist has asked me not to ask him questions!'

All of my patients say that greatly reducing questions, and rephrasing them, is the hardest part of all in Preventive Therapy. It is difficult to remember to do it and sometimes it is impossible to know what to say. If this happens, don't worry about it, just put it in question form. However, for most of the time, with practice, people can think of a way of saying what they want to say without it being a question. 'What do you want for your supper tonight?' can easily be changed to, 'We're having fish and chips tonight and I think we'll have peas. You will like that, I think.' 'Have you washed your hands?' becomes, 'Don't come for supper until you've washed your hands' or, 'Let me see if you have washed your hands.' 'Have you put your toys away?' can be replaced by, 'You will have to put your toys away now'; 'Do you know where you put it?' becomes, 'Let's try to find it' and so on.

For a question that would require a longer answer it is sometimes more difficult to substitute it with a non-question. But, for example, instead of, 'Tell me all about the party, what did you do all that time?' one could say something like, 'I would love to hear all about the party; perhaps you will remember to tell me when we get home.' Thus you are leaving Benjamin free to talk about it if he wishes but you are not putting any pressure on him to speak.

Some types of questions will put Benjamin under more stress than other types. One which requires the simple answer 'yes' or 'no' may never produce a stammer and, if this is so, it is quite safe to ask those questions.

When the subject of conversation is of *his* choice and appears to be an invitation for you to ask a question, that may also be safe. For example, 'Mummy, do you know what I would like to do today?' invites the reply, 'No, what would you like to do?' Questions, where the subject of conversation is the choice of other people, are much more likely to produce stammering.

Any question requiring an explanation is to be avoided if possible as uncertainty will reflect itself in speech.

Questions that are threatening in any way and which

therefore cause him stress, are your invitation for him to
stammer. 'What did you do *that* for?' implies that you are
annoyed with him and puts him in a position where he has got
to think of a reason or an excuse.

Even more devastating is a question that *accuses him* of
being responsible for some misdeed, '*You* did that, didn't
you? You broke that plate. Now tell me the truth, you did,
didn't you?' It is far preferable to tell Benjamin that you are
very cross with him and why you are cross, and leave it at that
without making him try to explain. It makes it so much easier
for him at this time in his life when he needs speech to be as
easy as possible. You may expect plenty of stammer-free
years ahead when he can be required to explain his
misdeeds!

After a little while – in fact, within just a few weeks – you
will find that everything begins to fall into place. Once
learned, it becomes natural to ask only a few questions and
you will find that you no longer have to concentrate very
much. Questions, put in non-question form, become a way
of life.

What can be done about other people asking questions

Regarding questions put to Benjamin by people other than
his parents, or the adults in that household, the parents really
need to decide for themselves what is the best thing to do,
under their particular circumstances. Clearly, you cannot ask
a shopkeeper to stop saying, 'Which sweets do you want?' or
someone in the street from saying, 'And how are you today,
Benjamin?', but you can easily tell friends and relations, if
they talk regularly with Benjamin, that you are stopping asking so many questions because it increases his stammer, and
would be very grateful if they could do the same. You can
explain by giving them examples of what to say. Similarly,
young children in the family could not be expected to cut
down their number of questions, but older children might be
expected to do so. You should certainly have a word with
Benjamin's teachers if he is at school and explain to them
what you are trying to do and that you would be very glad if
they would also try. Direct questions, when the teacher

points at Benjamin for an answer, should certainly be avoided. Indirect questions, when the entire group is asked 'Who knows the answer to this?', are not a problem because answering then is voluntary.

The results

Let us now suppose that every adult who talks more than just a little with Benjamin, has virtually stopped asking him questions. His parents, in particular, have put a lot of hard work into it and have cut down dramatically, perhaps asking six or seven a day instead of a hundred. Other people cannot be expected to concentrate on it so fully, nor share the parents' concern, but they too have got into the way of not asking Benjamin questions very often. This procedure has probably taken about one month. Now what happens? What has already happened? What may parents reasonably expect as a result of all the efforts they have put into helping their Benjamin?

First, you may be sure that Benjamin prefers it as it has greatly reduced the pressures that, in the past, were put upon him to speak. I would be very surprised indeed if the stammer had not decreased to some extent but I would be equally surprised if the stammer had entirely disappeared. Anything between these two extremes would not surprise me. The vast majority of parents I see report a considerable decrease in the stammer, but this does not necessarily happen within a month – it could take two months. Whatever the degree of improvement, if there is some, it is wise to continue with the strategies you've adopted. If there is *no* change in the stammer after, say, two months it would be pointless to continue with the same degree of concentration, but, nevertheless, I would not return to the old pattern of asking questions 'all the time' on the grounds that asking questions *is* a pressure on speech and we want to remove all possible pressures. This is for the child who does sometimes stammer when you ask him questions and the stammer shows no signs of improving even when you have greatly reduced the number of questions you ask him, but clearly would not be relevant for a child who never stammers when he is asked a question (very rare).

One mother who, with her husband, had worked through the Umbrella therapy of not reacting negatively to the stam-

mer and then the therapy of greatly reducing the number of
questions, came into the clinic and said, 'Before we start on
anything else, I want to tell you that Jeremy's stammer has
gone, well almost gone. It started disappearing as soon as we
stopped asking questions; it is two weeks since I saw you and
Jeremy has hardly stammered on a single word since then.
The change is so extraordinary we can hardly believe it.'
Delighted as I was, I had to tell this mother that stammers
never disappear altogether in just a few weeks and that she
was not to be surprised or disappointed if it took quite a long
time to overcome it totally, and that there would surely be
ups and downs on the way. There always are, but you can
cope with them if you know what to do. It is worth saying
more about this little boy who had made such a dramatic
improvement.

A case history

Jeremy
Jeremy, who was four, had been a quiet boy and always very
well behaved: he held his Mummy's hand, did as he was told
and never drew attention to himself. During the first weeks
that we were using the Umbrella therapy his stammer did *not*
decrease. There were, however, changes in his behaviour,
and they were very important changes. He had stopped giving up speaking altogether and saying, 'Never mind, it
doesn't matter' when, previously, about once a day, he had
said this when the stammer became severe. Very soon after
this his mother noticed that he was becoming generally more
confident and independent. He was beginning to volunteer
information, to say rhymes aloud spontaneously and to
imitate a dancer he had seen on television, saying, 'Look at
me, look at me!' – he had never done any of these things
before. In addition, his nursery school teacher remarked that
he had stopped getting huffy. His parents were surprised to
find that Jeremy was standing up for himself and even
becoming quite cheeky, which greatly pleased them because
previously he had never said 'boo' to a goose. They said he
was now '. . . a real boy for the first time ever.' These were all
encouraging signs of improvement in self-esteem but,
although they had all occurred within a few weeks, the stam-

mer itself had remained unchanged. At that point we started the reduced question therapy and then the sudden and massive improvement in the stammer occurred.

A few weeks later, however, his mother said to me, 'His stammer is terrible – not as bad as when we first came but it is very bad again.' It turned out that Jeremy had been into hospital for treatment of an ear condition and that was when the stammer returned.

In Preventive Therapy it is rare, as I say, for a child to go on improving steadily without any setbacks. Almost anything that substantially upsets the child in any way is enough to cause this. However, if the child has been making progress, then the setback is only *temporary*, so don't worry about it. Special holidays, accidents, being ill, being tired, being afraid, starting school, changing schools, are frequent causes of temporary setbacks. It is typical for these to last only a week or two before the stammer begins to pick up again. It may be a month, however, before he gets back to his former level of improvement.

Some points to remember

Before proceeding to the next chapter I would just like to emphasize some aspects of the reduced question therapy that will need your concentration.

You will be surprised at the number of questions you ask Benjamin! In the early stages of reducing them it would be useful, for one day, to make a note of the questions you ask, then, at the end of that day, go through them to discover how many questions you asked and also how many of them were necessary. A week later, repeat the exercise so you can find out what progress you have been able to make.

It is difficult, in the early stages, to remember to reduce the questions. When you do remember, it is often difficult to think of something to say instead of a question and it needs a lot of thought. If you just cannot think of something else to say, however hard you try, do not worry about it. It is better to ask the question and then, when you have a quiet moment, think about what you could have said instead. We do not want to be absolutely rigid about it or give up asking questions altogether as we are only trying to remove one specific pressure from Benjamin's speech. Some parents find this therapy quite fun and also very interesting to do, especially when they see the rewards it usually brings. They also say that they feel much more relaxed as a result of cutting down questions. Once again, I suggest that you should feel you are managing adequately before moving on to the next stage of Preventive Therapy.

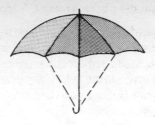

CHAPTER 4

Demanding speech

Sometimes the removal of just one or two or three pressures is sufficient to send the stammer on its way out. It may be that the Umbrella and the reduced question therapy have so greatly reduced Benjamin's stammer that it has almost disappeared. If so, this is excellent. Either way we shall proceed with the removal of another specific pressure, that of demanding speech. But first, let's take a short break. It is probably better for Benjamin not to have too many sudden changes in his environment because changes tend to make little children confused and even insecure. For this reason, if you and the other people in your child's world have made several changes in behaviour towards his speech, you will all benefit from not making further changes straight away. I suggest that you continue with your present therapy but wait for a week before adding to what you are already doing.

When your week is up and you begin working on the Preventive Therapy of *not demanding Benjamin to speak*, you will probably find it short and simple compared with what you have done so far. I know that I ask much of parents but I also know that they are very pleased to have something positive to do and very relieved to see the changes in Benjamin's speech.

Much of what I suggest means postponing some of the disciplines you would normally apply to Benjamin's upbringing. Parents always worry about discipline; I care about it too but I care much more about the stammer. When discipline is a pressure on speech, however, it should be delayed until some months after the stammer has gone. What are the options? If you insist on discipline for speech you may well have a child who will stammer for life. If you postpone discipline for speech, say until the child is six instead of four, you may well, and most probably will, have a child who outgrows his stammer. Put so bluntly there is little choice. Preventive Therapy involves postponing disciplines that involve speech.

'Say' and 'tell'

When you demand speech you not only tell Benjamin that he has got to speak but you also often tell him which words he has got to use. Usually, but not always, you start with the words 'say' or 'tell'. For instance, commonly you will say such things as:

'Say hello'
'Say goodbye'
'Say please'
'Say thank you'
'Say you're sorry'
'Say that rhyme for Aunty Mary'
'Tell granny that story'
'Tell daddy what happened at nursery today'
'Tell me where you got that biscuit'
'Tell that joke to John', and so on.

All these demands for Benjamin to speak need to be stopped; you should never require Benjamin to 'say' or 'tell' anything, not even to 'say his prayers'. There is no need for him to say 'hello', 'goodbye' or 'please' – they do not matter. If he does not spontaneously say 'thank you' on occasions when you think it does matter, then you can thank the giver on his behalf, it is easy. If Benjamin is with you it is quite sufficient to say, 'It was a lovely present you brought for Benjamin, thank you very much.' If you are not within his hearing you may wish to add, 'I'm not making him speak while he has this speech problem.' If you wish him to say he is sorry, instead tell him that you are cross with him, for whatever reason, and tell him not to do it again but refrain from telling him that he has to say something.

Parents, particularly mothers, like to show off Benjamin by telling him to say a rhyme or recite a piece of poetry he has learned or, as we mentioned before, tell a story or tell a joke.

They may also be so delighted when he produces a long or difficult word that they exclaim, 'Say it again, say it again', but Benjamin should never be congratulated for saying long or difficult words nor asked to repeat them. Preventive Therapy asks that you never attempt to show off his speech; it is a totally unnecessary speech pressure.

If you gain pleasure from asking him to 'perform' ask yourself why. The answer may well be that you are proud of him and want to show other people what a clever chap he is. It is natural for parents to feel proud of their children but, when one has a stammer, any exhibiting of his speech talents must be avoided. Somebody aptly said, 'Speech is primarily a tool, not an ornament.' Of course, if Benjamin tells jokes or says rhymes spontaneously that is different because *he* has then made the decision to speak and he chooses his own audience, which is not at all the same as you telling him what to say and to whom to say it.

Other times you may demand speech

Demanding speech does not occur anything like so often as asking questions, so it is comparatively easy to remember not to do it, especially as it so often occurs with sentences that begin with 'say' or 'tell'. Nevertheless it is possible to demand speech without the use of these two words when you require him to speak but may not actually tell him which words he has to use. For example, 'Benjamin, come and speak to granny on the telephone' or when you compel him to confess guilt, '*I* saw you pull the dog's tail; what a horrible thing to do. You have got to tell me why you did that and promise me that you will never do it again.'

It is probably impossible in a normal household to be one hundred per cent aware of the times you demand speech. Nevertheless, whilst you are putting Preventive Therapy into practice, you become more and more aware of it, and this helps you to eliminate it progressively. You may, for example, be playing the game of I Spy with Benjamin. You are saying, 'I spy with my little eye something beginning with T'; after a few ums and ers Benjamin suddenly says, 't t t teddy bear'. At that moment you realize that you have demanded speech. If other children are also playing the game even more pressure is put on Benjamin because he wants to be the one with the correct answer and he also wants to be the one to get the word in first, so he will feel the need to speak quickly. The same problems may occur in any word or guessing games. Naturally, if such games do not cause him any anxiety or stammer then there is no point in avoiding them.

You may also unwittingly demand speech if you have not understood Benjamin's words and you ask him to repeat what he has said. It is preferable not to ask him to repeat at all as this frequently causes stammering. Instead you may be able to guess what he has said or even just smile in acknowledgement. If this does not satisfy Benjamin it is up to him to say it again or to put you right by saying something else, if that is what he chooses. It is particularly important that you do not ask him to repeat what he said if he stammered whilst saying it or if he has been unable to complete saying what he set out to say.

Parents usually find that not demanding speech is comparatively easy to get used to. Nonetheless it does take concentration and practice and it means you need to be on your guard against saying certain things, even though it is much easier not to have to think about what you are going to say. Parents, intent on their child being well behaved, automatically seem to tell him to 'say' something. There have been several occasions when I spent half an hour with parents discussing the need to stop demanding speech in all its detail and, after their child had joined us for five minutes' play before leaving the clinic, they went out of the door and the mother either said, 'Say goodbye' or 'Say thank you'! It only goes to show that habits are not broken in half an hour!

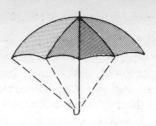

CHAPTER 5

Interrupting

If Benjamin's stammer has now apparently gone, or nearly gone, you may ask, 'Do we need to continue with further Preventive Therapy?' The answer is 'yes', it would be wise to do so. It may be that Benjamin is just having a 'good patch' when stammering almost disappears for a period of time but does not mean that he will not have further episodes of stammering in the future. If the stammer does not return within a few months the signs are very hopeful but you cannot be sure that it will not then return within the following few months. In my experience nine months of fluency must be maintained before one can say with confidence that the stammer has been overcome. Therefore, during the first months of fluency, or near fluency, it is a sensible precaution for you to be aware of what other speech pressures exist so that you can remove them and thus create an even better chance of the stammer not returning.

In discussing the speech pressure of *interrupting* I am going to ask you not only to *stop interrupting Benjamin* but also to *allow him to interrupt you*. Discipline is not going out of the window, it is only being temporarily postponed.

We must all know at least one adult who speaks incessantly, prattling on and on with a seemingly never-ending flow of words, scarcely stopping for breath. Any feeble attempt we make to interrupt only makes the speaker raise his or her voice, to drown ours, and carry on oblivious to any desire on our part to join in the conversation. This type of speaker has aptly been termed a 'verbal vulture' because the incessant speaker constantly interrupts but makes sure he or she is not interrupted. Heaven help Benjamin if he has such a parent.

The chronic interrupter makes us stop speaking, forget what we were saying and stops us listening to what is being said because we are trying to remember what it was that we had started to say. He or she finishes our sentences for us, often incorrectly, shows impatience with what we are saying and tries to stop us starting to speak so that he or she can speak instead. Such people make conversation difficult and unpleasant for fluent adults let alone a disfluent child. If you happen to be one of the few mothers or fathers who speak or interrupt in this manner, you will need to hope very hard that Benjamin is one of the three per cent who outgrow their stammering spontaneously and not the one per cent who only outgrow stammering with the correct help.

Most of us, however, share our conversations in a more or less reasonable way and it comes naturally to us to take turns in speaking and to scarcely notice the occasional interruptions. But there is still a tendency on the part of parents to behave as though it is all right for them to interrupt their child, sometimes repeatedly, whereas they think it rather rude to be interrupted by him. This step in Preventive Therapy takes account of the parents' feelings of not being altogether happy about allowing Benjamin to interrupt them, although they usually agree that they ought not to interrupt him. But once they have put the therapy into practice and found what a difference it makes to Benjamin's stammer they are only too willing to carry on allowing him to interrupt.

The effect of interruption on Benjamin's speech

Every time you interrupt Benjamin, whether or not he is stammering, it means that he has to start speaking again and, as we have already seen, stammering occurs most frequently at the beginnings of speech, which means that you are behaving in a manner that is likely to increase the stammer. Interrupting is also likely to cause him frustration and make him feel that what he has to say cannot be very important because you are not interested in hearing what it is – such feelings are enough to make anybody more hesitant than usual. In addition he will feel that he must speak quickly to get in what he wants to say before being interrupted again. The pressure of time, the feeling that it is necessary to speak quickly, is one of the commonest causes of increase in stammering, yet parents, unknowingly, subject their stammering child to this pressure over and over again, and, at the same time, they are saying, 'Benjamin, for goodness sake slow down!' No wonder he gets confused!

Difficulties you may experience when putting this therapy into practice

Learning to stop interrupting Benjamin takes a little getting used to. In the early stages you may interrupt unintentionally and then kick yourself for doing it but it just takes a little while to learn. As with other steps in Preventive Therapy, parents can help each other achieve their end by the occasional smile, raised eyebrow or whatever knowing look helps most. There was one occasion when it was necessary for a little four-year-old boy to be present in the clinic while his parents and I were discussing the interrupting therapy. I could see no reason why he should not be present because he was aware of his stammer and there was no particular secret about what we were discussing. The little chap played happily on the floor whilst we talked, apparently engrossed with the toys and unaware of what we adults were talking about. However, on their next visit, his parents laughed heartily because, they said, 'If we interrupt by mistake Benjamin says, "The speech therapist told you not to interrupt me"!' Even though this may seem a little patronising, it does show how important it was to Benjamin that he should not be interrupted.

I do not think it is reasonable to expect any parent to stop interrupting entirely. A child is never a verbal vulture but he may well be a chatterbox, and no parent can tolerate being unable to say certain things at certain times. It is important to cut down as much as you possibly can and it is especially important that you do not interrupt him when he is talking to himself. Children often live little parts of their lives in a world of fantasy and they talk to themselves, completely fluently, as they act out whatever is in their minds. In these moments of creativity and fluency it would be completely unjustified to break the spell.

When I ask parents to let Benjamin interrupt them they have all sorts of legitimate reasons why he should not do so: 'but he interrupts *all* the time', they say; 'It sounds so rude, especially when we have friends in, whatever would they think of us?'; '*I* don't mind if he interrupts but his father hates it; he doesn't think Benjamin should have everything his own way.' Despite these objections, believe me, it *is* necessary. Benjamin has a stammer and we want him to grow out of it so when he has something to say we don't want him to have to stop to think 'is it convenient to speak now?', we want him to just speak. It is a pressure on his speech to ignore him or 'ssh' him. Therapy is only temporary and you will find that allowing him to interrupt you is very easy once you have made up your minds to allow it.

Parents can be genuinely irritated by interruptions from their children, particuarly if they occur frequently and especially if husband and wife are trying to have a serious conversation. Therefore, I ask parents to keep their serious conversations for the evenings when Benjamin is in bed, if at all possible, and they are then free to talk in peace. Any topic that calls for an uninterrupted period of time is more suited to the hours when Benjamin is not around. Admittedly allowing interruptions can be trying for parents, but it soon becomes a habit and it pays dividends. I have never yet known parents who regretted allowing their Benjamin to interrupt.

Although no parent could realistically be expected to allow one hundred per cent of interruptions, you cannot go half measures in Preventive Therapy. The parents of one little girl Jane, who was five years old and had a severe stammer, assured me that they had already been advised to allow interruptions and had been doing so. 'But', they said, 'It would be impossible to *always* let her interrupt; she interrupts *all* the time. We don't mean just a lot of the time, we mean literally hundreds of times per day. She never stops.' I asked them if they were willing to try, as an experiment, letting her interrupt hundreds of time per day, just for the three weeks until their next appointment. They bit their lips whilst they tried to assess whether this would be possible. 'Yes', they agreed, 'Let's give it a try. We'd do anything to help but we will just have to see how we get on.' That was more than enough for me. Three weeks later they returned.

'Jane's stammer has almost gone', they said, 'It's incredible; we would never have believed that letting her interrupt us could make such a difference, and it was far easier to do than we expected.' Jane's father went on to say, 'The stammer hasn't gone altogether, but what we now think of as a "bad day" means that she has stammered just a few times; a few weeks ago we would have considered that a "good day". We feel sure now that she will get over it.'

Jane's parents no longer considered allowing her to interrupt as just an experiment. They had already decided to carry on with Preventive Therapy for as long as necessary.

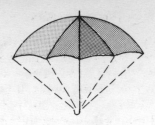

CHAPTER 6

Giving attention

It makes a tremendous difference to how Benjamin feels about speaking if, when he talks to you, you listen to and are interested in what he is saying. Parents should be the kind of people their children enjoy talking to. When the telephone is ringing, the baby is crying, the cat is trying to get in by the back door and Benjamin is pulling at his mother's clothes saying, 'Mummy, mummy, mummy', how are we going to apply the Preventive Therapy of *giving attention*? Essentially, our task is to listen to Benjamin but at the same time we must recognize that it is not practical to listen carefully all the time to a talkative child.

When we speak we want the person to whom we are speaking to listen to what we are saying. If what we are saying is a bit complicated or difficult to explain it helps us if we feel assured that the listener will wait for us and not make what is already difficult even more difficult. If the listener's attention wanders we become aware that what we are saying is not interesting enough to hold his attention. It is not a pleasant feeling. Benjamin has added difficulties in this situation because he is likely to be more non-fluent if he does not feel free to express himself without being in any way hurried or embarrassed. Inattention, half attention or attention lost half-way through his conversation is likely to decrease his confidence and increase his stammer.

Hearing and listening

Hearing is not the same as *listening*. When we hear the birds

singing or children playing in the street or a train drawing in
to a station we know what is happening, we hear what is happening, without really paying attention – we are hearing but
not listening. When Benjamin speaks, it is easy, it may even
be a habit, to passively hear him but not actively listen to
what he is saying. Perhaps he wants to tell his mother about
some event he has just witnessed while she is watching television and she pays little attention to him; 'Mummy, mummy,
mummy,' he says, but she does not respond although she is
aware that he has spoken. Alternatively, she may stop to listen
but speak rather impatiently saying, 'What is it Benjamin?'
Either way Benjamin will feel that he had something exciting
to tell his mother and she was not interested. Any such rebuff
will do little for his self-esteem and even less for his
speech.

There are all sorts of reasons for parents not listening to
what their child is saying. It may be that he seems to talk
incessantly, that his parents think he has little of importance
to say, that they are too busy to listen, that he always seems
to talk just at the time his mother is having to concentrate on
something else, that his parents are just too tired, or too
bored, to listen. We often listen just sufficiently to hear, or
half hear, what is being said while we continue what we are
doing, or we may stop what we are doing but feel rather
annoyed because of the interruption and resume our task as
soon as possible. We may, on occasions, be so engrossed with
our own thoughts that we are only aware of when the talking
stops or we may even deliberately switch off mentally until
the talking stops so that we can then get on with our own
thoughts or activities again.

Listening carefully does not seem to come naturally unless
we make a special effort, so that, for example, we can hear
someone who has been having a conversation with somebody
make the remark, 'I pricked up my ears when I heard that',
which must mean that, although she was listening, she was
not originally giving her full attention to what was being said
until something of particular interest came up. But Benjamin
needs help, he needs *our* help and we need to make that special
effort for him. When Benjamin speaks he tells us something
about himself which he wants us to understand. He uses
words to convey his message but he also uses them to tell us
about his thoughts and feelings. It is important for us to

understand the meaning hidden behind the words he speaks. When he tells you that he has lost his ball he is not only telling you that he has lost his ball but he is also asking you to come, to come now, to help him find it. When he tells you that he has hurt his finger he is also asking you to kiss it and make it better again. Words are only the tools he uses to tell you how he feels. Sometimes he seems to think that actions speak louder than words. We must all, at some time, have seen Benjamin pulling desperately at his mother's skirt, trying to get her attention. If she does not give it to him he will eventually say something, most probably stammering from sheer frustration. Parents sometimes say, 'I wonder if he stammers on purpose; at times I think he does. He'll do anything to get my attention; he stamps his foot, pulls at my clothes, screams and stammers like anything.' If Benjamin has to work so hard to get attention it is certainly time he got it and he must be in very great need of it. To a child who needs it, a little attention is better than none at all. If he can get his parents' attention only by stammering he cannot be blamed for using his stammer and he should not be put in the position where he needs to use it to advantage. It is perfectly possible, and natural, that he may start off speech with a stammer if he knows that is the only way to make his parents listen to what he wants to say.

When putting the therapy into practice is not so straightforward

Other parents say that listening to Benjamin does not present a problem, that they enjoy listening and talking with him and believe that they almost always listen carefully and respond appropriately. Much depends upon the individual parents and their particular child. If he is not too demanding, his parents may listen to him as easily as they listen to each other. Sometimes, though, they find it more difficult to listen to Benjamin if he is stammering a great deal because they find that the stammer distracts them. When this happens it is helpful for parents to train themselves to concentrate on their own ears instead of their child's mouth, so that they listen to what he is saying and not to how he says it.

Nevertheless, to be asked to give full attention to Benjamin every time he speaks, both when he is stammering and when he is fluent, is clearly unreasonable if not impossible and if he is a very talkative child this is particularly difficult. There must be a practical solution, not a compromise of half-listening all the time but a *method* of listening carefully only when necessary. Let's talk about the possibilities.

Preventive Therapy rests on the premise that Benjamin is quite capable of understanding that he cannot be given immediate attention in every circumstance. His parents should make this clear to him *at the time* of the event when giving attention is inconvenient. They should also tell him when they will be able to listen to him. For example, if Benjamin demands attention at the time that his mother is feeding her baby, she could say, 'I'm feeding the baby so I cannot listen carefully to you at the moment. I shall be about half an hour and then you can tell me what you want. I will tell you as soon as I am ready.' As another example, suppose that Benjamin's father has just come home after a busy day at work and collapses in an armchair. Benjamin jumps on his knee demanding fun and games, which his father cannot tolerate just at that moment. He can say, 'I'm tired; I want to sit down in peace with a cup of tea and read the paper. I do not want to talk or play just now; we will have a game after supper.' Such explanations will teach Benjamin, if he doesn't already know, that sometimes it is necessary for him to wait. This should not increase his disfluency because he knows where he stands and will understand the reason why he must wait. It will not make him feel badly about himself or his speech. Nevertheless, one should only postpone giving attention when there is a legitimate reason. Foisting Benjamin off without explanation must also be avoided, for example, 'For goodness' sake leave me alone' will not only make him feel rejected but gives him no *reason* for leaving you alone and will not satisfy Benjamin. It is not the same as knowing that you are tired and that you will play later.

If Benjamin is a chatterbox you need some method that will give you some freedom from attending to his almost perpetual chatter. First let it be said that many little children, the ones who talk all day, often talk to themselves; they neither intend nor wish their parents to listen to them. As parents, you know very well when Benjamin is chatting thus, and there is no call for you to listen. So, *learn to listen selectively, learn to interpret the signs.* As you observe Benjamin you will notice that when he wants your attention he does certain things as a way of sending you signals to make you understand that he has something important to say: perhaps he just comes and stands close by you or tugs at your clothes or raises his voice or is more non-fluent than usual – perhaps he stammers. He will have his own particular way or ways of impressing upon you that he wants you to listen carefully. When he comes specifically to *you* he clearly wants to say something that is important to *him*. At these times you should always listen to what he wants to say.

One mother told me that when her daughter wanted to speak to her she always said, 'Let's go and sit on the sofa while you tell me about it.' This is an excellent idea because it shows the child she is getting her mother's full attention and it also shows her that she has as much time as she wants.

We have already said that many children who stammer have 'good days' and 'bad days'. When Benjamin is having an almost fluent day you should go out of your way to give special attention to his speech and create conversation as additional speaking on these days will reinforce his fluency.

Failing to give attention to Benjamin's speech, then, is clearly a pressure in that parents say, 'His stammer increases if we don't listen to him' or, 'His stammer decreases when we listen to what he says.' However, compared with the removal of the other speech pressures we have discussed, I cannot recall a single instance of parents having put this principle into practice, returning to the clinic and saying, 'The difference in his speech is amazing; the stammer has almost gone.' Perhaps, nowadays, more parents *do* listen attentively when Benjamin talks than they did in bygone days when it was expected that little children be seen but not heard.

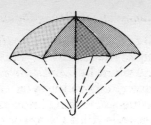

CHAPTER 7

Competing for the chance to speak

Benjamin's stammer may be expected to increase when he has to compete for a chance to speak. There will be times in his life, probably daily or even several times daily, when he finds that other people begin to speak at the same time as he begins speaking and, owing to other people speaking excessively, he is unable to break into the conversation. These occasions are particularly likely to occur when there are other children in the family, although Benjamin may also find that from time to time he speaks, or tries to speak, in competition with his parents.

When two adults begin to speak simultaneously, one of them usually stops speaking to allow the other person to speak first. However, when an adult speaks at the same time as a child the adult may assume that she has the right to continue with what she was saying, ('Be quiet, mummy's speaking') and that the child should wait until she has finished. When two children speak simultaneously, one may give way in favour of the other, or both children may continue speaking together, regardless of the fact that they may not be properly heard or understood.

As much as possible, *Benjamin should be protected from having to compete for an opportunity to speak*. To bring this about, his parents will have to watch themselves, watch each other and enlist the help of the older children in the family. Family life will make it impossible to give Benjamin full protection but his parents and the older children should be aware that people do compete for speech and, preferably, they should be prepared to minimize Benjamin's frustration by allowing him to speak first. On the other hand, if such preferential treatment is considered unfair by the other children, it would be reasonable to work out a system whereby the children take turns in speaking first on the occasions when they wish to speak at the same time. For, if the other children do not willingly allow Benjamin to speak first, he will be liable to interruptions from them. He will also be liable to time pressure as they convey to him, either by body language or by words, that they want him to get a move on. If the other children are forced to allow Benjamin to speak first they may make it clear to him that they resent it. 'It's not fair', they may say, 'you're always allowed to be the first because you stammer.' Thus, there is the danger that Benjamin could be made aware, or more aware, of his stammer. This would be far more emotionally damaging to him than having to wait for his turn. Taking turns, even if frustrating, is fair.

Typical situations when Benjamin will be competing for the chance to speak

Mothers sometimes tell me that when the children arrive home from school together they are so full of news that they all speak at once. They also tend to speak at the same time when they have shared the same experience. Perhaps they have seen something very funny on television, a spider in the bath, an accident, been invited to a party – whatever it is, they all want to be the first to tell their parents the news. It is on such occasions that Benjamin needs his parents to come to his rescue and ease him out of a threatening situation.

Competing for the chance to speak can also occur when people are speaking one at a time, but one or more listeners are eager for the speaker to stop speaking so that they can speak instead. At the first pause in the conversation someone will jump in quickly to say something, even if the original speaker has not finished what he or she set out to say.

Meal times, when families usually get together, can be difficult for Benjamin. When everyone else can enjoy airing their news and views to a captive audience, Benjamin may become aware that he cannot speak like the rest of the family, especially if he gets left out altogether. A talkative family

having a lively discussion, perhaps as they sit round the table
over a meal, could easily fail to notice that Benjamin has not
been given a chance to speak throughout the entire meal.
There have been no pauses long enough for him to join in. If
he has attempted speech he has probably got no further than
an initial stammer that has gone unnoticed by the rest of the
family. A family discussion at any time can make speech
difficult for Benjamin if he is not given sufficient time to
speak and he should not be put in this position. Other family
members are able to seize the conversation by jumping in
quickly and the loudest and the quickest children are likely
to be the first to get attention. Parents should be on the
lookout for this, be aware of their own speech habits and
avoid getting carried away with adult opinions or problems
that make them take too big a share of the time.

When you are implementing Preventive Therapy and the
family is talking together, Benjamin must have his fair share
of the time. He need not have more than his fair share, but he
should have enough time to make his contribution to the conversation so that he does not feel left out. He must know that
there is sufficient time for him to speak – even if he chooses
silence rather than speaking he will know that he has had the
opportunity to speak. I do not suggest that he is given an
allotted time but rather that there should be breaks during
the general conversation when the family give him a chance
to speak by remaining silent themselves.

One mother told me that she was puzzled because her
small son, Gary, always stammered more in the evenings and
at the weekends than at other times. 'It's a funny thing', she
said, 'as soon as the older children come in from school he
begins stammering. It can't be their fault because they never
"correct" him or take any notice at all of his stammer.'
Nevertheless, it appeared that Gary's increase in stammer
was associated with the presence of the older children. 'Do
the older children talk a great deal?', I asked, 'Oh! They never
stop', she said, 'They talk all the time.' Gary scarcely stammered when they were at school, but in the evenings and at
the weekends, when they were at home, he was having to
compete for a chance to speak and this was noticeably affect-
ing his stammer.

No family, particularly where there are other children, can
altogether avoid competing for chances to speak. However,

being aware that competition exists makes it possible for parents to control it to a large extent. This will greatly reduce, if not eliminate, this pressure on Benjamin's speech. Frequently, family members agree to let Benjamin speak first. Failing this, parents try to ensure that their children speak one at a time and also take turns in being the first to speak. Families manage the problem by their own particular methods and what suits one family does not necessarily suit another.

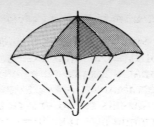

CHAPTER 8

Pronunciation and grammar

The onset of stammering occurs most frequently at just about the same time that a child's language development peaks. This is surely not a coincidence. As the child's use of language develops, he uses more speech sounds, more words, longer words and longer sentences. In addition he tries, all the time, to use his new words correctly and also to put them in the correct sequence. He is learning one of the greatest of all skills, the acquisition of language. With so much to learn, and to reproduce, it is clear that the child, during the process of learning language, will pronounce many of his words differently from adults and he will use shorter sentences and a different grammatical construction of sentences than those adults use. It is also clear that many normal non-fluencies will occur as the child produces, hundreds of times daily, an ever-growing vocabulary and flow of words. It is not surprising that non-fluencies are the norm rather than the exception.

During this period of learning his native language, it is important for a child to have a good speech environment, which is one with plenty of speech stimulation, but in the simple sort of language that he can understand and learn to copy. He should be allowed to learn language at his own rate and not be subjected to the pressure of being required to make certain sounds, say certain words, or put words into a particular sequence. Usually, normal speech and language will develop spontaneously, given that the child has enough simple language to listen to, and a warm and loving environment in which he enjoys speaking. But, this may well be the time when the child's non-fluencies seem so excessive that you begin to wonder whether or not he is stammering.

If you suspect that he may be developing a stammer or if you are almost sure, or sure, that he is developing a stammer, it is extremely important that his attention is not brought to his speech in any way whatsoever. Even if parents are not making Benjamin aware of his stammer, they may call attention to his speech in other ways. This will make him aware of his *speech* so that he will eventually become aware of his stammer. If his attention is brought to deviations in his pronunciation and grammar, he will begin to put effort into speaking. When putting Preventive Therapy into practice, therefore, a child who stammers *must be allowed to speak without correction of his pronunciation or grammar*. Any corrections are pressures on his speech.

Things you can do to put this part of the therapy into practice

Anything you do or say that draws Benjamin's attention to his speech will, in time, make him aware, or more aware, of his disfluencies. Anything that makes him feel that his speech is not acceptable as it is, will make him feel that speaking is less, rather than more, pleasurable than it used to be. Anything that makes him feel more hesitant about speaking will decrease his confidence and increase his disfluencies.

When a little child says his first words his parents are delighted regardless of the fact that he is not pronouncing them correctly. If, for example, he points to a car and says 'tar' his parents will exclaim, 'He said car!' At a later age, however, when his parents judge that he should be pronouncing his words correctly, they may say, 'Don't say "tar", say "car"'. These parents do not appreciate the fact that if Benjamin has not yet developed the sound 'c' he is unable to say 'car' so they are asking for the impossible. Benjamin, in his early years, may well substitute several speech sounds with the other sounds that he has at his disposal. Thus, instead of saying, for example, 'Susan got my bike', he may say, 'Tutan dot my bite'; he is pronouncing his words in his own way. It would not adversely affect Benjamin's stammer if you should occasionally repeat his mispronounced word with a correctly pronounced word. When, for example, he says 'tar' you could simply say, 'Yes, there's a car.' If he says, 'Ice pudding', you could say, 'Aha; it's rice pudding.' These responses do not imply that you wish him to say words the 'right' way, they simply offer a stimulus that he will automatically copy when he is ready.

Similarly, when Benjamin's sentence construction is immature, his efforts should not be corrected; do not change his sentences by trying to make him put them into adult form. Neither should progress be met with delight from his parents lest he should feel that high speech standards are exceedingly important. His language will, to a large extent, be influenced by the language models around him. You should therefore avoid rapid changes in conversational topics, which he may find confusing. Also to be avoided are speech patterns that are too complex and a continuous flow of words, because Benjamin may feel that he ought to copy these and, being unable to do so, become more hesitant than usual.

A sentence such as, 'Daddy is coming in at six o'clock and we have to be ready because we are all going out immediately after he comes in' is far too long and complicated. A more suitable form of language would be, 'We must get ready now; we are going out with daddy.' Even the condensed, 'Get ready; going out' would be preferable if Benjamin understands that more easily. He needs language models in keeping with his own language development so that he finds speech easy, not something out of his reach.

Benjamin's sentences will not be grammatically correct. As with the pronunciation of words, parents tend to expect errors early in Benjamin's life but, as time progresses, they judge that he should be speaking differently and that he needs help in using the correct words and putting them into the correct sequence. Thus when Benjamin says, 'Me going out' his parent will say, 'Not "me", *I'm* going out.' When he says, 'Where you go?' he gets the response, 'Not "where you go", where are you going?' John accuses Benjamin of not giving him his half share of the sweets and Benjamin replies, appealing to his mother, 'I did, didn't I not?' and so on. While applying Preventive Therapy, his grammar must not be corrected as such correction is a speech pressure.

Correcting grammar comes so naturally to some parents that they may easily correct it without thinking, although they had intended not to. If this is the case, it may take a week or two to get into the habit of disregarding the grammar. Benjamin needs to feel free of anxiety when speaking, so he needs to be free from all speech correction, he needs to feel that speech is easy and effortless and he needs to feel free *at all times* to take all the time he needs to get his thoughts sorted out and to decide which words to use. It is more important for a child to enjoy speaking than it is for him to speak with the proper pronunciation of words or the correct grammar. So, be permissive with your child's speech.

Coping with a second speech difficulty

Occasionally a child will have two distinct speech problems: a stammer and something else. The question is whether or not this child should receive speech therapy for the second speech disorder. Any direct speech therapy (as against indirect therapy through play with the child, or therapy via the parents, such as counselling) will make the child aware of his speech and therefore constitutes a speech pressure, which may increase the stammer. When Preventive Therapy is being given to a child it is preferable that he be stammer free for nine months before treatment is given for any other speech disorder. This view stems from the fact that, if a child does not overcome the stammer he may well have a problem for life, that this disability can be and often is, enough to spoil his entire future. Chained to anxiety about speaking, he may grow up to avoid people, avoid situations, feel inferior to other people and wish, as so many adults do, that he had been given appropriate help when he was young.

In the clinic where I work we postpone speech therapy for second speech disorders until the child has been free of his stammer for nine months and find that this works out very well. It only means that the child whose speech is not always easily understood or whose language is a little delayed, waits a year or so before specialized treatment is given for his particular second speech disorder. The difference is that he overcomes his second disorder by the time he is six or seven instead of, say, five years old, which is a small price to pay compared with possibly having a stammer for life.

This said, sometimes the second speech disorder is serious and requires immediate and long-term speech therapy. In such cases the speech therapist, after taking a careful, detailed, case history to determine the priorities, will be able to make a professional judgement in deciding which course to take.

A stammer may be *caused* by the presence of the second speech disorder. If the second disorder is causing the child much emotional stress it is possible for a stammer to begin as a result. Treating and alleviating the second disorder would relieve the stress about speech and thus, indirectly, also relieve the stammer.

CHAPTER 9
Taking stock

We have now finished outlining and discussing the six specific pressures on Benjamin's speech. If you have been putting Preventive Therapy into practice in the ways described, I am sure that you will have found a tremendous change in Benjamin's speech and that, probably, the stammer has been overcome. Do remember, however, that the entire therapy programme may take anything from three months to a year, depending on how long it takes you to manage to remove the pressures and on how quickly Benjamin responds.

Getting back to normal

A few weeks after Benjamin's stammer has been overcome, or almost entirely overcome (if he, for example, only stammers very briefly on two or three words per week and he shows no anxiety when these few stammers occur), it will be time to begin getting back to normal. Every child is subjected to speech pressures and Benjamin now needs to begin to be treated in the same way as other children – he needs to get used to the pressures again.

Getting back to normal involves reintroducing the six pressures on speech, but a little at a time and one by one. I suggest that you follow the same order that you did when you removed the pressures, but first, a word of warning: do *not* reintroduce any pressure that causes any return of the stammer. You can begin this process by asking Benjamin an occasional question then, if all goes well, you gradually increase the number of questions until you feel that you have reached a normal number. Remember that any *sudden* changes in Benjamin's environment may cause him to be confused or troubled, so he needs plenty of time to come to terms with any changes. Perhaps a period of about two weeks should be devoted to the reintroduction of each speech pressure, but, obviously, take it a bit more slowly if two weeks seems to be too sudden for Benjamin.

After you have reintroduced questions, begin demanding speech once again, gradually building it up until you feel that you are doing it quite naturally. If Benjamin still shows no sign of stammer as a result of what you are doing, proceed to interrupting him occasionally and, from time to time, let it be known that it is not convenient for him to interrupt you. When the time comes, begin to reintroduce the other pressures, namely, not always giving him the full attention that he wishes for when he is speaking to you, allowing some competition for the chance to speak, occasionally correcting his pronunciation and grammar if you think this necessary and if it is helpful. When you are reintroducing these six speech pressures it is extremely important to notice if they produce any stammering. If they do, you should postpone reintroducing them until they do not cause any return of the stammer. It is also important to remember that we are all normally non-fluent. When Benjamin has overcome his stammer he may still, at times, repeat sounds, syllables and phrases but these normal non-fluencies are always completely free of tension and of anxiety.

When the six speech pressures have been reintroduced and are at a level that is normal for your household with no return of the stammer, the time will have come for you to forget about speech and all the efforts that you have made on Benjamin's behalf. Getting back to normal may take approximately three months. Then, after a further six months of no return of the stammer you may consider that, except under very exceptional future circumstances, the stammer has been totally overcome.

What to do if Benjamin is still stammering

If Benjamin's stammer has *not* yet been overcome and you

therefore have not yet reintroduced the six speech pressures, there may be other pressures still on him. These would not be specific speech pressures but rather those that affect his speech *indirectly*. It is to these that we will now turn our attention.

PREVENTIVE THERAPY PART TWO
The indirect pressures on speech

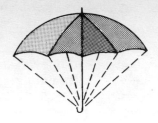

Chapter 10

Expectations

It is not the intention of this book to advise parents on how to bring up their child. All of the suggestions made relate only to how fluency may be either directly or indirectly influenced. When I see parents in the clinic we talk about the same things that you are reading about in this book. However, during our meetings, other topics frequently arise and the conversation then turns to these topics. They fall mainly under four headings:

- the expectations that parents have of their child
- the discipline they use
- other possible communication stresses
- questions that parents ask.

These topics are discussed in this and following chapters.

If Benjamin is persistently frustrated or bewildered in his life he may continue to stammer even though, using the methods described so far, the specific speech pressures have been removed. We cannot expect fluency from a child who is, for example, frequently over-stimulated and excited, nor from a child who has constant doubts about himself or who is frequently frightened or humiliated. All such emotions are likely to disrupt fluency and cause stammering, particularly if he speaks during the times that he is affected by these emotional states. Pressures that adversely affect Benjamin's feelings will indirectly affect his speech. His feelings will be partly determined by the expectations you have of him.

The Umbrella symbol sits at the beginning of this chapter as a reminder that the therapy of not reacting negatively to the stammer, and the virtual removal of the six specific pressures on speech, should still be in force. In addition, *your expectations of your child should be realistic and reasonable*.

Encouragement is good for Benjamin, it will help him to achieve and achievements will increase his self-esteem, in turn probably lessening his stammer. Nevertheless frustrations arise when parents keep on expecting their child to achieve things that he is not yet capable of achieving or when they are unreasonable in their demands.

The importance of realistic expectations

Benjamin will begin to have self doubts if your expectations are too high, regarding both his *behaviour* and his *achievements*. Expectations should therefore be within his limits and not make him feel that he is unable to measure up to them. Perfectionism should be avoided because it only brings with it stress and makes a child feel that he can never do well enough. Parents who are constantly discontented with the best that their children can do are probably insecure themselves. They need to understand their own motives. If *they* have failed to achieve, they, perhaps, then try to gain through their children what they feel they have not managed to achieve for themselves.

Children suffer from numerous unnecessary frustrations when parents expect too much of their behaviour. 'Boys don't cry', they say to a boy who is crying or, 'Don't be a baby.' 'Keep your clothes clean', they say to a child who is enjoying himself playing, 'I don't expect a child of your age to make such a mess.' Such comments may make Benjamin feel obstinately frustrated because he finds nothing wrong with crying or getting dirty. He may be expected to manage all sorts of tasks from tying his own shoe-laces to looking after a younger child. Conversely, he may be frustrated by not being allowed to perform the tasks that he thinks he can manage. 'You can't wipe the dishes' his mother may say, 'You're too young, you may break them', or, 'Let me do your buttons up, you'll only get them wrong.'

When there are differences of opinion like this it would be wise to *talk* with Benjamin about his behaviour so that he understands how you feel and you understand how he feels.

This way, differences can be ironed out. As a result you might both agree, for example, that boys are as liable to tears as girls and that old clothes should be worn for getting dirty in. A great many problems can be overcome by discussion and it is much more satisfying for a child to be encouraged to have his say than it is for him to be issued with commands without explanation.

Parents do sometimes seem to expect their children to be models of good behaviour. They are expected not to touch anything in a toy shop, to sit still when told to do so, eat what they are given, do as they are told and leave household articles where they belong. Obviously children have got to learn what is socially acceptable and what is not, yet sometimes they are denied the most harmless activities, often only for the sake of tidiness. A houseproud mother will tell her child to put the cushions back on the sofa just when he has made them into a train on the floor; a fussy mother will tell him to stop playing with the sugar bowl when he is busy building sugar castles. Benjamin thinks she is *always* saying, 'Don't do that', 'Don't touch that.' Not only does she seem to like things to be untouched and tidy but she also likes everything to be constantly clean – clean hands, clean face, clean knees, clean clothes. All sorts of little frustrations can add up to make a child's life generally frustrating and they are often things that are totally unimportant. Not being allowed to touch a hot oven is one thing, not being allowed to touch a cushion is quite another. When you are applying Preventive Therapy it is best not to be too fussy and not to expect more of Benjamin's behaviour than is consistent with his age and development.

If your standards are too high, not only his behaviour but also his achievements are bound to fall short: 'That's a funny man you've drawn, his arms are longer than his legs'; 'You should try harder'; '*Mary* is not afraid of the dark and she's only a baby'; 'You can do it if you think about it'; 'It can't hurt very much, it's only a scratch'; 'You managed to read it for me so you should have been able to read it for granny', and so on, and so on.

Parents may also make their child feel inadequate by comparing him with his brothers and sisters, the neighbours' children, or what the neighbours say about their own children. There is often a child next door who is made out to be quicker and brighter than anybody else. Anything that makes Benjamin feel ashamed, a failure, humiliated or that he has let his parents down, will cause the frustrations that increase the stammer. When you expect something of Benjamin you might first ask yourself if he is going to be able to manage it or whether you are expecting more than he can cope with.

We live in a culture that is competitive so we want our children to be as good as other children or, preferably, better. We want them to shine and win. We want them to make good impressions. In order to give their child a head start, many parents urge them to achieve and to go on achieving. This may be all right for some children, but if a child is unable to reach the heights expected of him he will feel a failure and his parents will feel disappointed.

One day a successful business man came to the clinic with his wife and son. 'Carl has a stammer', he said, 'and often he says his words badly so that we cannot understand what he says. I want him cured of both. I've made my own way in the world, I've worked hard and I want Carl to do the same. He will never be a success if he cannot speak properly. I have high academic expectations of him.' Carl was three years and nine months old! This father did eventually come to understand that it was premature to be thinking about academic expectations before the child had even started school. Fortunately for Carl he overcame both speech problems in due course, so even if he grows up under paternal pressure at least he will be fluent and pronounce his words correctly. Dealing with Carl's stammer was left to his mother, as his father deemed it 'woman's work' and she dealt with it admirably, making sure that all the speech pressures were removed and gained a perfect result.

Overcoming frightening experiences

Sometimes a child will appear to have almost outgrown his stammer, or may have stopped stammering altogether for just a few months and then he suffers a severe shock and the stammer returns, perhaps really badly. This may happen when a child has been badly frightened or has suffered any other serious emotional shock. We should not expect children who are only recently fluent to maintain fluency under such traumatic conditions but, then again, a recently fluent child will not necessarily begin to stammer again under such conditions, but he *may* do so. Anything, therefore, that frightens Benjamin should be avoided as much as possible. He may be a little frightened of certain activities, such as going into the sea or riding a bike or being expected to pat a dog. He may be frightened by certain people or scarey stories or television programmes. He may be frightened of certain conditions such as being left alone or having his bedroom door closed or going to bed without a light on. Usually these minor fears can be avoided or, better still, overcome with time and patience but without ridicule. Terrifying experiences, however, are not so easily avoided. They are usually events that occur without warning. An instance of this is when one little boy, Sam, had just started going to school and decided he would like to go home. He was unfamiliar with the large building and wandered through long corridors before he found his way to a back door. Outside was a busy city road. Somehow Sam managed to get to an island in the middle of the road, but he was unable to get off the island because cars were speeding in both directions. He was rescued but he was speechless. When he began to speak again his stammer had returned.

Avoiding over-excitement

Excessive excitement should also be avoided for it, too, can be responsible for a return of the stammer. One Christmas, Steven was not expecting very much. He and his mother lived alone and she had financial difficulties. That particular year she decided to make Christmas really wonderful for Steven, trying to make up for the few previous years when she had been unable to give him a real treat. She saved for months and bought him all sorts of wonderful presents. A real bicycle, football clothes and a football, a cowboy outfit and a radio, as well as smaller toys and sweets. Steven was shocked. 'He just stood there', his mother told me, 'He stood there with his mouth open, not saying a word. He hardly spoke that day. Next day his stammer had returned.' Deep emotional experiences, even pleasurable ones, affect speech and we should not expect it to be otherwise.

Social situations

Finally, some parents, whilst accepting their child's stammer at home, become embarrassed when he stammers in a social setting. Sometimes they feel that their child has let them down, sometimes they feel that the stammering is somehow a reflection upon themselves. Parents have often told me that they cannot help feeling embarrassed in a public place, such as a supermarket or when travelling on a bus, they feel that everyone within hearing distance is listening to the child's stammer and is judging the parents. One embarrassed mother said to me, 'It is such a let down. The children are so intelligent. They are good looking and smart. We look like the ideal family until Michael opens his mouth, then when he stammers it is as if everything collapses.' Some parents can't help feeling a degree of shame about their stammering child.

Many people get embarrassed at times by quite trivial events, but it is better to accept and expect occasional embarrassments than to worry about them.

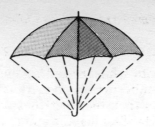

CHAPTER 11
Discipline

Sometimes parents say that they believe stammering in their child is just a bad habit, that he could stop stammering if he really wanted to and that he does it deliberately to be irritating. To any parents who believe this I would say, 'Try doing it yourself and find out if you are as clever as your little child.' It is impossible to stammer consistently on particular sounds, with a particular degree of tension, in a particular manner, unless the stammer is real. Stammering arises from a lower level of consciousness than conscious intention. It is not a deliberate act, although it may appear to be. 'Benjamin cannot get his own way', parents sometimes say, 'so he stammers.' It is much more likely that Benjamin cannot get his own way and becomes frustrated so that, in fact, it is the *emotional frustration* that causes him to stammer. If you believe that Benjamin is stammering deliberately you are at risk of reacting negatively to it, possibly by attempting some sort of discipline, and any discipline regarding speech should be avoided. Appropriate general discipline, however, will minimize the emotional frustrations that cause stammering.

The speech problem we call stammering has never been fully understood and attempts to stop it by force have never been successful. In the Middle Ages stammering was regarded as a personality disorder and it was believed that sufferers were possessed by the devil. The 'possessed' person was given vile concoctions of garlic and vinegar to drink to make him vomit and thus purge out the devil. Incredible as this now seems, it is not so very long ago that a child might have got his face slapped for stammering, be isolated in a room or be told that he was not to talk until he could talk properly.

Punishment

These days stammering is probably only rarely deliberately punished since the bringing up of children has become more and more permissive. Nevertheless, the child who stammers is still frequently 'punished' for stammering even though it may not be intended to seem like that.

Ridicule, irritation and impatience are all punitive and even praising or rewarding fluency is an indirect punishment because it implies that fluency is welcome but stammering is not.

Coping with your own feelings

Sometimes parents feel guilty because their child stammers. They think that they must have done something wrong in bringing him up. The truth is that stammering will occur in the best of all possible homes and families *and* it will occur in 'bad' homes, in the same way that behavioural problems arise in children whatever their background and no matter how hard parents try to avoid them, for not all children are little angels. Sometimes one child in a family is clearly different from the others, despite an almost identical environment and upbringing. Sometimes he is excessively jealous of a brother or sister or he may be extreme in his demands for attention. He stands out as the rogue. However excellent the parents, he can be moody, destructive, defiant, quick-tempered, jealous, bumptious and so on, presenting his parents with problems that are difficult to cope with. There must be a reason for such behaviour but explanations are not always easy (or even possible) to find. Fortunately these forms of behaviour are usually intermittent and they tend to occur as phases which some children go through but grow out of. Fortunately too, we love our children because they are our children, not because they are perfect. Unacceptable behaviour from Benjamin, while a cause for concern, should never lead to unacceptable behaviour from his parents – he should never be made to feel unloved.

It is important to remember that *the relationship between parents and child should be loving and warm but, at the same time, general discipline is necessary, which should be consistent and based on reason. Lack of discipline, inconsistent discipline and unreasonable discipline lead to emotional frustrations that cause or increase stammering.*

A child who stammers needs a loving and warm relationship with his parents, one that increases his feelings of security and confidence and that takes particular account of how this relationship will affect his speech. We return once more to how Benjamin *feels* about himself.

Why some approaches to discipline can be harmful to Benjamin's speech

Everybody knows what a loving and warm relationship should be like but, if a child has a stammer, it is easy to damage that relationship by thoughtless remarks instead of developing and maintaining conditions in which the child's speech is never criticized and in which conversation runs freely and spontaneously. Freedom of speech requires as few rules as possible. The tendency to stammer is increased by criticism of speech in general. Comments such as, 'Don't talk so much', 'Don't ask so many questions' and, 'For goodness' sake be quiet' are belittling and harmful. Disapproval too, of what Benjamin says specifically, is likely to make him more hesitant. However, parents have their own standards and Benjamin must understand that there are limits. For example, there may be a few rude words, such as swear words, that you will not allow him to use, but it is best to forbid as few words as possible. Sometimes words are tabooed for no good reason. A child may, for instance, call his grandad 'gramps' and will be corrected, 'That is rude, you must call him grandad.' Likewise, parents may be offended by their child speaking in his local dialect – 'Don't speak like that', they say – or by him making a statement of fact, such as 'I don't like granny' and come back with the retort, 'You're not to say that.'

Parents, quite unwittingly, or for the sake of 'standards' that are, really, unnecessary, may interfere with their child's speech and cause him to be uncertain, making his attempts at speech tentative and lacking in confidence. Benjamin wants the approval of his parents and so takes notice of what they say. If high speech standards are set, he will try to keep up with them. Unable to manage, he may then begin to react against the high standards by avoiding speaking situations – particularly if he is already finding his stammer symptoms unpleasant. When he wants to speak, but at the same time fears to speak in case he meets with disapproval, a conflict arises that will cause his speech to become more hesitant and less spontaneous.

In an environment that lacks love and warmth, where speech is criticized and restricted, Benjamin may well feel himself to be a small appendage to the family, unrespected and unsure of himself. Alternatively, a loving and warm environment will allow him to feel that he is a respected and full member of the family. Uncriticized, free to say what he wishes, free to have emotional outbursts, free to express his feelings and thoughts without inhibition, he will be allowed the spontaneity of speech that goes hand in hand with confidence and promotes fluency.

In a generally permissive speech environment the few words that are forbidden can easily be dealt with by explanation followed by strict adherence to what has been agreed.

General discipline is necessary

All of the requirements in Preventive Therapy mean that there is a total removal of discipline so far as speech is concerned. However, this is only temporary and is reintroduced at a later stage, after the stammer has been overcome (see Chapter 9, page 76). A child who stammers gains security from knowing that his speech will not produce a threatening situation, but he will lack security if there is no discipline to limit his general behaviour.

We all need to feel secure, otherwise we are under stress and fearful of what may happen to us. Knowing that we can dial for emergency services if we need them, that we have a bit of money in the bank, that we have a house to live in, that we have enough food to eat and so on, all give us a certain feeling of security. And we also feel more secure by recognizing that there have to be some rules in society that limit our behaviour: we would not want to drive without a highway code or play tennis on a court without boundary lines.

Benjamin, too, needs to feel secure, secure in the knowledge that there are limits to his behaviour, limits to what will and what will not be tolerated. He will trust his parents because of the loving and warm relationship and, in trusting them, he will come to understand that necessary discipline is for his own good. If a child is not disciplined to a sensible degree, he will not only create havoc in the household but he will be confused within himself and un-respected by other people.

Children seem to respond readily and willingly to a certain amount of discipline – not the now outdated variety of discipline that was discipline for its own sake, but that which makes it clear that enough is enough, that they can go so far and no further and, if they do go further, there will be consequences. They need to know that if they act in a certain way there is a price to be paid.

Such discipline is essential for an ordered society and for an ordered family. It gives a child a sense of social awareness and, above all, security. Most children experiment by testing the water, seeing if they can 'get away with it', but if the consequence is punishment they soon learn to conform with the family rules. A child accepts the consequences of nature and respects them – if he has a hard fall he may expect a grazed knee, if he touches the cooker he may expect burned fingers. In a similar way he should be able to accept from his parents the consequences of misbehaviour. Knowing the limits makes growing up easier for Benjamin, certainties are easier to accept than uncertainties.

The type of behaviour that merits punishment, and the manner in which that punishment is meted out, depends upon the attitude of the particular parent involved. One mother may feel that an appropriate response to Benjamin, if he bites someone, is to bite him back, while another may smack his bottom and another may give him a good telling off. Parents have their own standards and make their own rules. It is to be hoped that the rules are necessary, sensible and few but, whatever the case, like the other members of the family, Benjamin must conform.

Some family rules are more necessary and sensible than others. Forbidding speech at mealtimes and having to remove shoes upon entering the house, for example, are clearly less appropriate disciplinary measures than not being allowed to play in the road or to touch electrical appliances.

Untidiness is a frequent cause of arguments. Perhaps excessive tidiness makes the difference between a house and a home. A *house* has always got to look perfect in case somebody calls whereas a *home* is where children can grow up in a relaxed way. I once had a patient who was thirteen and had stammered since she was three. She had daily battles with her mother because she made the whole house untidy and particularly her bedroom, which her mother said was a disgrace. It was littered with clothes, her mother could not tell the clean from the dirty, books and records were all over the floor and, 'She hadn't even got the decency to put toffee wrappers in the waste-paper basket.' After much discussion and some firmness I persuaded them to reach a compromise. The daughter was to put her dirty clothes in the bathroom to be washed and was to keep the rest of the house tidy, but her own bedroom could be as untidy as she liked, including the toffee wrappers on the floor. The daily battles stopped, the stammer quickly showed signs of improvement and, within a few months, had almost totally disappeared.

If Benjamin has not been subjected to discipline (occasionally parents are nervous of disciplining their child because, if he has not been used to it, they find it increases his stammer) and if you believe that you ought to discipline him, it is best to introduce the changes gradually. Children become confused and uncertain by sudden changes. When disciplining your child it is always advisable to be firm but approach the situation in a matter-of-fact, kindly way without emotion – being firm does not mean being cross. It is also best not to keep him in a state of suspense. For example, if you say 'we will do this' or 'we will not do this', he knows where he stands whereas saying 'we will see' will make him feel uncertain, hoping something will happen but afraid that it will not.

If Benjamin *has* been used to having his own way with little or no discipline, even if you introduce it gradually, you can expect that he will fight for what he has had in the past and continue in his attempts to control his parents and the situation. You should also be prepared for a phase of increased stammering during the period in which his demands are not met. If a child controls the household the likelihood is that he will continue to stammer because he is insecure. The situation is unnatural and the home is likely to be chaotic rather than calm. If he has to go through the process of learning that he does not control the household and that 'no' means 'no', you may expect the deterioration in his stammer to be followed by an improvement once he has come to terms with his changed environment. This can be a very trying time for parents as they witness Benjamin's stammer worsening and wonder if they are doing the right thing. Eventually, though, Benjamin will respond to the discipline, so long as the parents do not weaken in their resolve, and he will emerge more secure and almost certainly with a much decreased stammer.

A definition of the word 'discipline' is 'the maintaining of order among those in one's charge.' With children, order is usually achieved in one or more of three ways:

● verbally, by the use of reason or instructions
● by deprivation, for example, disallowing favourite edible goods such as sweets and ice-cream or not allowing the child to watch television or cancelling outings and so on
● by physically hurting the child by smacking.

One does not need a sledge-hammer to crack a nut and it seems reasonable that, whenever possible, verbal instruction should be the first means of instilling discipline. Punishment by deprivation is rather more drastic but may be necessary and sometimes more effective. Physical punishment, except for the small, quick smack, in my opinion, should only be used after warning the child that a smack will follow if he refuses to conform. Parents should never do anything that *frightens* their child. I have known of parents who have locked their child in a room as punishment when they knew he had a fear of being in a room with the door shut, and of a mother who deliberately frightened her child by threatening to leave home so that he would be left all alone. Adults should be able to control their children without resorting to such despicable behaviour.

Discipline should be consistent

Parents use discipline to stop their child running riot and

behaving in an unacceptable way, to aid in the promotion of a calm and ordered household and to train the child to gain a measure of self control. The parents are the managers and, if their discipline is to be effective, they need to be consistent in their management.

To be consistent the parents need to agree with each other (avoiding, for example, the mother saying that the child should have a definite bedtime and the father saying that he should be free to go to bed when he feels like it) and to apply the discipline they decide on consistently. Benjamin cannot accept that bedtime is at a given hour if his parents are not in agreement over it. When parents cannot reach agreement it is best to arrive at an understanding whereby they act together and put up a united front. It is essential that the discipline they use is the same or similar because Benjamin cannot be blamed for taking advantage of inconsistency – it is natural to do so. He must know where he stands so that he can learn what is allowed and what is not allowed.

Two case histories

Christopher
Four-year-old Christopher's parents did *not* put up a united front and he took full advantage of this inconsistency. His father did not believe in rules: 'Where I come from young children are not disciplined', he said. Christopher's mother tried to make rules but, because he had his father's support, Christopher was able to ignore them. This caused his mother much frustration and she got into the habit of shouting at him whenever he was naughty. He was *very* naughty, spending most of his time making her shout. He must have enjoyed a feeling of great power over his mother, he could make her behave in almost any way he wanted. One fairly typical day was when she made the beds and he immediately stripped them, she made them and he stripped them again. Then he threw every cushion on to the floor. She picked them up and he threw them down again. Then he began to paint the wallpaper. By this time his mother was screaming instead of shouting and, as she began to wash off the paint, Christopher went off to strip the beds again. His poor mother could not cope with this and she hit him. She felt bad about this and so she hugged him.

By the time her husband came home from work she was quite beside herself – worn out with shouting, frustration and despair. 'Christopher has been dreadful all day, he has not stopped being naughty, for goodness' sake take him OUT, get him out of the house for half an hour and leave me alone while I pull myself together', she said. So the father did as he had been asked, he took Christopher out. He took him to the shops and spent the half hour buying him toys!

Although this is a rather extreme example of what can happen when parents disagree about discipline, parents *do* disagree and the child can soon learn the art of one-upmanship. This is encouraged when the child's father says, 'You have been a naughty boy today, getting your mummy upset.' His motive is to scold but the result is a re-inforcement of the child's feeling of power over his mother. When a child is with his mother most of the day, only seeing his father for an hour or two in the evenings, it is natural that the mother should be more taken for granted than the father. If her discipline is supported and consolidated by the father, when he is at home, the consistency of approach will make the discipline much more acceptable to the child. He may argue but he will know where he stands. Without this combined approach the child's one-upmanship flourishes.

Alex

One mother said that her son, Alex, refused to go to bed unless she went to lie on his bed with him until he fell asleep. For the sake of peace she agreed and she thought it would be quicker to get Alex off to sleep before preparing the evening meal. One night she unintentionally fell asleep. When she awoke, hours later, Alex was not in the bed. She found him in the lounge, with her husband, playing snakes and ladders! If one parent persists in undermining the authority of the other, it is to be expected that their child will trade on their differences to achieve his own ends. Benjamin will be able to say, 'Daddy lets me do it' when his mother tells him to stop doing something. Children often use all their wits to get their own way. One way is to nag. If Benjamin wants something, and if there is any chance at all of getting it, he may well go on and on nagging at his parents until he gets what he wants.

If only parents would stick with what they have said in the first place Benjamin would engage them in fewer battles: 'I

just could not stand it any longer', they say, 'After saying
"no" a hundred times I finally gave in and said "yes." ' Such
confrontations are best avoided and, after all, parents are not
obliged to argue back.

It is wise to be consistent in responding to any antisocial
behaviour from Benjamin. If he sticks out his tongue, for
example, and one parent laughs but the other gets cross with
him, he will not know whether or not his behaviour is acceptable. Equally, he will not know if one parent laughs at such
behaviour on one occasion but gets cross with him on another
– their responses need to be predictable so that he can
anticipate approval or disapproval.

Discipline should be based on reason

A child is more likely to do what he is told if what he is told
makes sense to him. Once rules are learned they do not need
to be explained over and over again but day-to-day corrections may need explaining. Benjamin wants to know the
reason why. In fact, he is always asking 'Why?' and he should
be given satisfactory answers so that he can understand the
reasons why some discipline is necessary. When parents say
to him, 'That's naughty', 'Don't do that', 'That's rude' and so
on, he is likely to argue the point. Arguments are less likely to
arise if, instead, explanations are given. For example, 'It was
naughty to run out on to the road because you might have got
hurt', 'Don't throw your ball over the fence because the
neighbours don't like it' and, 'We don't use that word in this
house because it is a swear word.'

A totally unreasonable, but by no means unusual, conversation may go like this:

'You're not to say that'
'Why not?'
'Because it's naughty'
'What's naughty?'
'Don't be silly'
'I'm not silly'
'Yes you are'
'Why am I silly?'
'Because I say so.'

Parents sometimes use discipline without reason, because

'we have always done it like this' or they have copied perhaps
from their own parents or from the neighbours. If parents
cannot find the reasons for their own discipline it is little
wonder that they have to resort to such phrases as 'mummy
knows best'. Their discipline should make sense to themselves and to their child.

Conflicts between parents and child sometimes arise
because of bribes, threats, misunderstandings and broken
promises. 'If you are good I will give you some money to buy
sweets'; 'If you play quietly, while I have a cup of tea, I'll cook
you some chips for supper.' Was Benjamin good? Did he play
quietly? Parent and child may have different interpretations
of what is good and what is quiet and thus a dispute may
begin.

Conflicts can also occur when a child appears to be feign-
ing illness in order to get his own way or has unusual needs
that do not require discipline but medical advice. One such
child was always hungry almost immediately after meals, no
matter how much he had eaten. In these instances it is very
easy to discipline or even punish a child unfairly. In general,
children tend to speak less fluently when they have been
punished and particularly so if the punishment has been
unfair.

Parents can base their discipline on reason but, at the
same time, expect too much of their child. Nowadays we have
many two-language families among us. It is natural that they
should wish to maintain their own culture and their own
language in addition to the national culture and language, but
speaking in two languages may be more than a small child can
manage. One such child was able to speak very little English
but spoke Punjabi at home with his parents. When he started
school, where he was obliged to speak only English, he began
to stammer. We asked his parents to communicate with him
only in English, to stop speaking Punjabi in his presence
and not to react, in any way whatsoever, to his speech. We
suggested that their own language could be reintroduced at a
later date, if the stammer was overcome. In fact the stammer
was overcome within just a few months and it is almost certain that it had been caused by language-related stress.

However skilled parents may be in the use of discipline,
and in basing it on reason, there are certain to be times when
their child's behaviour goes beyond the bounds of for-

bearance. There are limits to how much parents can tolerate and, when they are driven too far, frustration and anger can take precedence over their usual responses and cause them to behave in a manner that is out of character. In my opinion this is of little importance so long as it is not a frequent occurrence. Parents are free to have emotional outbursts and should not feel guilty or embarrassed by them. When things have calmed down, however, it would be a reasonable gesture of reconciliation to tell Benjamin what happened, a statement of fact not blame, thus maintaining the loving and warm relationship. Benjamin may well be glad to know that his parents, too, are capable of reaching breaking point, capable of crying and that they respect him enough to be able to explain what brought it about.

We would have rigid, unreasonable homes if rules were never bent. Even in homes where rules are few and punishment is light there will be times when these are waived to suit the occasion. Exceptions to discipline are also based on reason: Benjamin may be allowed to go to bed later than usual because it is a special day; he may be allowed to watch television all day because he is unwell; he may be excused for sticking out his tongue because he had been wrongly accused when he did so, and so on. Furthermore, parents cannot be expected to put theory into practice all the time; they may forget or simply not bother or even not notice what Benjamin has said or done. If parents are confident that they are able to control their child they can afford to be flexible without fear of him taking advantage.

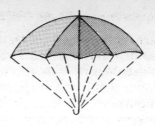

CHAPTER 12

Other communication stresses

Stress, we are told, is bad for us. However, we need a degree of stress. If we were totally relaxed, both physically and mentally, we would shuffle about like zombies without a thought in our heads. Without some physical stress and tension we would be unable even to stand or move, and without mental stress we would be unable to think, observe or be alert. It is the *unwanted* stress and the excess stresses that cause problems.

Like everyone else, Benjamin will have what I call a basic stress level, to which will be added greater stresses according to what is happening to him at any given time. The level of stress put on him will constantly vary and when it is high he will be more likely to stammer because stress is reflected in speech. As we have already discovered, stress can affect speech both directly, as discussed in Chapters 3 to 8 on speech pressures and indirectly, that is when the stress is not directly connected to speech itself, as discussed in Chapter 10, Expectations and Chapter 11, Discipline. There still remain any other stresses that disrupt fluency and which are personal to any particular child and these I shall discuss now.

Clearly, it is not possible to list every possible stress that a child may undergo or have to live with. Rather, I shall try to categorize the kinds of anxieties children may have and that may cause increase of stammer. Many stresses are just a part of everyday living that we cannot avoid (for example, being tired after a late night); other stresses we can reassure Benjamin about (for example, we can comfort him by assuring him that his grazed knee will not hurt for long), but Benjamin should be protected, whenever possible, from the more serious stresses that clearly have a detrimental effect upon his stammer.

Preventive Therapy rests on the principle that *if Benjamin's circumstances seem to be stressful it is up to his parents to be alert to the conditions that affect his speech behaviour and to take steps to alter the disturbing factors.*

Some other main stresses on speech

Let us now turn to some of the conditions that may raise Benjamin's stress level, bearing in mind that stammering may be expected to continue while the child is still under the influence of the stress.

Fears

For example, the dark, being left alone, punishment, animals, insects, television programmes, playground swings and slides, having his hair cut, being taken into the sea

Shock

For example, witnessing an accident, personal accident, losing a pet, sudden noise, being lost

Speed

Anything that causes Benjamin to talk or act quickly – for example, a sudden challenge, being made to hurry, impatient listeners, people talking quickly

Excitement

For example, outings, parties, going away on holiday, Christmas, birthdays, visitors, beginning nursery school or school, special occasions

Physical stress

For example, being ill, out of breath, tired

Uncertainty

For example, being unsure how to behave, being the odd one out, irregular routine

Authority figures

For example, doctors, dentists, teachers, policemen

Feeling of loss

For example, breaking a favourite toy, a friend leaving his street, death or departure of a close relative

Handedness

Making a child use his right hand when he prefers to use his left

Harmony in the home

It is obvious that a child will suffer some stresses if he is brought up in a home that lacks harmony. If, for example, Benjamin's parents argue a great deal, he will be affected by their behaviour. He will pick up on the tensions and may wonder whether he is going to be caught up in the crossfire. I recall one family where the parents were not on speaking terms and used their child to deliver written notes to each other.

Perhaps few families are without some tensions but any extremes in family conflict impair the confidence and security that help a child to overcome his stammer. Naturally, for some parents, relations are strained, but it should still be possible to prevent their child from feeling torn apart. To illustrate this I will describe how two families managed to protect their children when their marriages failed.

Two case histories

Mr and Mrs A

Mr and Mrs A had two little boys aged two and four. The two boys had quite severe stammers that had shown some improvement during the months when their parents started applying Preventive Therapy, but the improvement did not continue. In discussing possible stress factors with the parents, it transpired that they were considering divorce: they were unable to spend even a few minutes together without a row breaking out, resulting in recriminations, shouting and slammed doors. I asked the parents if, for the sake of the children's speech, they could possibly manage to postpone their rows until the evenings when the children were asleep, having written down all their topics of discord so that nothing would be forgotten. And I asked them to close the door so that the children would not hear their raised voices. They agreed to do this and conscientiously carried out the agreement. Finally they divorced but the children had been spared from the rows and both totally overcame their stammers. Five years later I happened to meet their mother in a shop and she said that neither of the boys had ever stammered again.

Mr and Mrs B

Mr and Mrs B had three children, one of whom stammered. They decided to separate but both agreed that 'the children come first.' The children lived with the mother but the father visited their home every day and spent as much time with the children as he wished; he was always made welcome. The little boy said to me one day, 'My mummy and daddy live in different houses' as if it was the most natural thing in the world. He totally overcame his stammer.

Children usually manage to take the small everyday stresses in their stride, but too many small stresses can build up to the point where they put a child under general stress. When this happens, or with the more serious stresses, it is not surprising if some stammer still lingers. Paying attention to the stresses, and striving to eliminate them as much as possible, may well tip the balance and bring Benjamin down on the side of fluency.

My description of Preventive Therapy and how to use it is now complete and I hope that it has been helpful to you. My great wish is that one day stammering will be fully understood and fully preventable and that this book will have been one positive step in this direction.

If you feel that you need support in working to overcome Benjamin's stammer, you should contact a professional speech therapist. You may wish to work through this entire programme with her help but, if you seek an alternative therapy for stammering, the advice given here should still be useful to you. Speech therapists may be reached through making enquiries to the District Speech Therapist via your District Health Authority, National Health Service.

CHAPTER 13

Questions parents ask

What caused him to stammer?

There are no clear-cut answers to the baffling problem of the cause of stammering. We know, however, that preventing it from developing in its early stages is much less of a problem than trying to overcome it once it has developed and become an established stammer. In pre-school children the onset of stammering is usually gradual, often with remissions, but with the symptoms increasing as time passes. When the onset is sudden, with more dramatic symptoms, this may be as a result of a traumatic incident but usually occurs in older children.

Numerous books have been written about stammering but they are written from different points of view and writers often disagree regarding the cause or causes. We have to consider that, particularly when there is stammering in the family, some parents will be more likely than others to notice their child's normal non-fluencies and suspect that he is stammering. As we have seen, once parents believe that their child is stammering they begin to react negatively to it and 'correct' it, thus making the child anxious about his speech. The seeds are then sown for a stammer to develop where there might not otherwise be one. Thus it has been said that 'the stammer begins not in the mouth of the child but in the ear of the parent.'

We also have to consider whether the child has a predisposition to stammer. We know that stammering frequently runs in families. It may be that a child, under certain conditions of stress, will begin to stammer because he is predisposed to do so.

Another viewpoint is that a child may begin to stammer because there is too much stress in his life – he can take so much and no more. Then comes the straw that breaks the camel's back and it is this last straw that causes his speech to deteriorate under the strain.

Many parents agree that their child comes under the category of one or more of these three possible causes of stammering, but there are still families where the child's nonfluencies have not been noticed or 'corrected', where there is no family history of stammering and where the child has never been under undue stress, although, as we saw in Chapter 1, it appears that it can be triggered off by events involving various degrees of stress.

If we carry out all the steps of Preventive Therapy will he get over the stammer?

So long as the speech pressures as set out in this book are removed and so long as the child feels secure and knows that his parents love him, my belief is that he will almost certainly outgrow his stammer. A peaceful and happy household may make it easier, but a home does not have to be ideal for a child to outgrow his stammer. Indeed, as we saw in Chapter 12, fluency can be achieved in homes that are far from ideal. It is worth reiterating that the speech pressures do need to be removed so that the child feels absolutely free of speech stress and they should only be gradually reintroduced after the stammer appears to have been overcome.

Year after year we see pre-school children overcoming their stammers – it is what we have grown to expect and there are few exceptions. Occasionally, however, there are exceptions. When a child is making progress but then suffers a traumatic event, the stammer may worsen or return to its former state. This is unfortunate but not a disaster because, within weeks or months, it usually picks up again. If, during this second period of improvement, another traumatic event should occur, the stammer may again revert or worse, this time take longer to improve. Then a third traumatic event may occur and the stammer, once more, reverts to its original state or becomes even more severe. By this time the child has not only suffered a great deal of stress but he is also a good deal older and, when he is older, a stammer is much more difficult to overcome. The importance of overcoming a stammer whilst the child is young cannot be overestimated.

It often happens that a young child will begin a period of stammering and overcome it by quite simple means, quite quickly. Sometimes, simply not reacting negatively to the stammer and greatly reducing the number of questions, as described in Chapters 2 and 3, is enough to stop the child stammering. Even so, I always go through all of the direct and indirect pressures on speech, with the parents, so that they are aware of them and thus able to reduce or eliminate them if the stammer returns. We have to remember that a stammer, in a young child, is frequently intermittent and it is thus quite possible to believe that the child has overcome it when, in fact, he is just having a 'good patch' but may begin stammering again at any time.

In carrying out the entire Preventive Therapy programme, it is important to work thoroughly and systematically through each speech pressure. In the clinic, with parents, we work through it in the order in which I have written it, but there are sometimes exceptions. If, for example, there appears to be a particular reason for the stammer, as with the child trying to cope with two languages mentioned in Chapter 11, that would obviously be our starting point or if, for example, there is clearly a problem with discipline, we would start there, but, in most cases, there is no conspicuous disturbing factor that one may suspect of being responsible for the stammer.

As we have said, parents usually need to change their attitude towards Benjamin's stammer. The ideas of not reacting negatively to the stammer and of removing the speech pressures, are new to them, and it takes time to adjust to the new regime. I find that parents want to go over the same points again and again and, for this reason, you may find it helpful to read the chapters two or three times, or more if necessary.

What will happen if he doesn't get over the stammer?

Remember that three out of four children outgrow their stammers spontaneously. If your child is one of the twenty-five per cent who does not outgrow it spontaneously, the chances are extremely high that he will outgrow it with Preventive Therapy. In the clinic we also see older children and adolescents overcoming their stammers through learning how to control stammering. Nevertheless, it is estimated that half a million people in Great Britain still stammer.

Stammering in its early stages does not show the vast variety of symptoms exhibited by the adult who stammers. As described in Chapter 1, the symptoms of pre-school children are almost always simple repetitions of sounds, syllables, words and phrases, prolongations of sounds and inappropriate pauses. These are much like those character-istics of normal speakers when under stress. We want to prevent a child from noticing the symptoms and, if he does notice them, we want to prevent him from reacting to them with anxiety. If he learns to react with anxiety it leads to him struggling to get the words out. Once the vicious circle is established – of anxiety about speech = stammer = anxiety about speech – the stammer feeds on itself.

The symptoms of stammering in young children are not only more simple but also much more consistent than in older children and adults. If a child does not grow out of stammering he grows into it – the stammer does not remain simple and consistent. As it develops, it increases gradually in frequency and severity. As the child grows older he begins to sense the interruptions in his speech flow and tries to stop them by exerting pressure on his speech muscles. The more he exerts pressure in his attempts to release the stuck words, the more severe the stammer becomes. If he continues, ever harder, to force the words out, this may eventually lead to accessory movements of the body such as jerking the jaw, tossing the head or stamping the foot. He finds, in his struggle to release a word, that the word is finally released when he, for example, jerks his jaw. He then attributes this release to the jaw jerk so he goes on using the jaw jerk when the words get stuck. Then comes the time when the jaw jerk does not succeed, so he finds another movement to release the word, for example, tossing the head. The jaw jerk does not go away at this stage but remains, along with tossing the head, as part of the stammer pattern. This is how stammer symptoms develop.

Many children are not greatly troubled by the fact that they stammer while, for others, it is a cause of constant anxiety, particularly if the stammer is severe and they get teased about it at school. The tendency is for them to worry about their stammer more as they get older. Adult sufferers, too, vary in their attitude towards it. Some regard it as somewhat inconvenient and wish it wasn't there, while some say that it has ruined their lives, reduced their personal happiness, made them fearful of social occasions and prevented them being successful in their careers. Others have a great deal of success in their chosen careers, but parts of their days are taken up with worrying about approaching speaking situations. Their pulse rate becomes rapid as they anticipate the meetings they must attend and the telephone calls they must make.

People who are not familiar with stammering have no idea what it is like to have a full-blown adult stammer. They think it is a small interruption of the speech flow, causing the speaker to feel vaguely inconvenienced and that sometimes it is done deliberately for effect. Little do they know. One well-known, fluent American speech therapist, who once had an extremely severe stammer, told me that, in his youth, he had spent two years on a farm as a labourer, pretending to be deaf and dumb so that he did not need to speak at all. One of my patients once took seven minutes to say the four words, 'Thank you and goodnight.'

A severe stammer can be very marked indeed. One sufferer wrote, 'I do not know the feelings of a person defaced by a burn or a scar, but I imagine them quite like the feelings I had, at first, about my tongue's new and unwelcome capacity.' When a stammer is very severe, even if the speaker does not feel that his life has been ruined, he feels frequent shame and embarrassment and believes that the listener will think he is thick because he is unable to talk.

The person with a fully developed stammer presents a complex picture of behaviour and attitudes. Stammers vary according to the situation. When he feels at ease, perhaps with his family and friends, even the most severe stammer may disappear and he will be fluent or almost fluent. Other situations cause him untold problems: certain people are difficult to talk to, telephoning and shopping may be difficult or even impossible. Some speaking situations may be avoided and in some situations he stops talking altogether. He fears specific words or specific sounds or he may find all words potentially dangerous. He begins to scrutinize words before uttering them. He worries about which sound the word begins with, how long the word is, where it comes in the sentence, and whether he can change it for another word. He tries to replace his fears with other attitudes, using techniques that he thinks will allow him to speak without stammering. He may adopt an aggressive attitude, one of confidence or one of humour. He may use gesture to distract himself and his listener from his speech. He may speak very rapidly, making all the words run together, so that he doesn't have to contend with the dreaded first words of sentences. He expects all kinds of reactions to his stammer. Whether his expectations are real or imaginary, he anticipates rejection, laughter, embarrassment and impatience from his listener. He wishes that his stammer showed, before he opened his mouth, so that he would not have to face that dreadful moment when he discloses that he is verbally impotent.

The intensity of feeling that some sufferers experience is, fortunately, not felt by all. There is much variation in how people who stammer evaluate themselves and their listeners.

Why do so many boys stammer compared with girls?

This is a question that has intrigued speech therapists since they began working with people who stammer because it became glaringly obvious that far more boys than girls stammered. Investigations have resulted in suggestions being made, but there are no conclusive or convincing explanations.

Different studies give different ratios, but this is to be expected because they have been carried out in different cultures, in different parts of the world, on different age groups and so on. According to published estimates however, on average, there is a ratio among people who stammer of about four boys to one girl.

People have hypothesized that:

- there is a male genetic predisposition to stammering
- because there is a greater susceptibility in males to most childhood diseases, stammering can be viewed as reflecting the vulnerability of the male constitution
- boys tend to compare unfavourably with girls in physical, social and language development and are prone to more difficulties in general speech and communication
- there are, perhaps, greater environmental pressures on boys. They are often less sheltered than girls and thus meet more competition leading to frustration and insecurity
- there are differences, too, in parental attitudes to boys and girls. Boys are generally expected to be manly, not to cry, not to show emotion
- it is possible that the male child has a less stable neuromuscular control system for speech, during the early years of his life.

Why does he stammer on some days but not on others?

The intermittent nature of stammering in some young children is not really understood, we only know that it happens. Sometimes they have days with little or no stammer and sometimes longer periods with comparatively little stammer, which may last several days or even weeks. As the child overcomes the stammer, the 'good patches' tend to get longer and the 'bad patches' get shorter. Because our knowledge on this aspect of stammering is limited we are at present obliged to accept, as a fact, that children may be much more fluent on some days than on others.

Laying aside the puzzling phenomenon of periods of near fluency, or even fluency, it would be a good idea on the days when stammering is clearly more evident than on average days to check through all the direct and indirect pressures on speech, just to make sure that you have reduced or eliminated any possible stresses.

What is the difference between stuttering and stammering?

These words are interchangeable and there is no difference in their meaning. Either term is used, although 'stammer' is usually preferred in the UK. In the USA 'stutter' is always used. People sometimes think that particular symptoms constitute stuttering and that other symptoms constitute stammering but this is not so.

How long will it take Benjamin to get over his stammer?

It is not unknown for parents to be given an appointment at the speech clinic and then, in the brief period before the appointment, for them to cancel it because their child is no longer stammering. They would be advised to still keep the appointment to discuss their child or, failing that, to contact the clinic again should the stammer reappear. On occasion, a stammer can disappear quite suddenly.

Many children begin to stammer in their ordinary life situations and no cause can be found or possible causes be suspected. If you think you know the cause of the onset of your child's stammer and if that cause is still there, removing it may bring an almost immediate cure, particularly if the stammer has only recently started. If, however, the child has been stammering for some time, perhaps six months, removing the cause may or may not be sufficient to remove the stammer. The cause may be quite easy to remove (for example, by stopping teaching the child to speak a second language), difficult (for example, if there is ongoing parental conflict) or impossible because it is no longer there (for example, if the child was hit by a car.)

Asking how long it will take for a child to get over his stammer is really impossible to answer. It takes as long as it takes so predictions have to be tentative. It will take longer for a child to overcome his stammer if he suffers a major setback as a result of illness or shock, for example, or a series of minor setbacks such as may result from repeated and prolonged periods of excitement or frustration. In the absence of these, and provided that Preventive Therapy for pre-school children is put into practice conscientiously while the child is still of pre-school age, I would expect some improvement within weeks, a marked improvement within months and for the stammer to have been overcome or virtually overcome within about a year. Sometimes it is overcome well within the year. As we have said, a further nine months of fluency is the real test and before this time has passed one cannot be fully confident that the stammer has gone.

Is there much research into stammering?

There was an ancient theory that stammering was due to a physical defect of the speech organs (muscles and so on that are used when we speak) and, over two thousand years ago, Aristotle declared that it was due to a fault in the tongue. So great was his influence that, as comparatively recently as 1850, some surgeons were still trying to treat stammering by cutting away portions of the tongue!

Scientific research into stammering began in the 1920s. As a result our knowledge about stammering is increasing. We are coming to understand better how to prevent it and what to do about it, but there is a continuing need for more research so that methods of prevention and correction may be increasingly more effective. Thousands of books and articles have been written about stammering and numerous suggestions put forward as to its causes, its nature and how it can be treated. Some theories have been investigated over and over again. For example, there have been over two hundred studies on the question of handedness, arising from one theory that training a left-handed child to be right-handed caused stammering.

In summarizing several hundred significant research investigations into the nature and cause of stammering, Bloodstein* states:

'Stammering** is predominantly a disorder of childhood, more common in males than females.

The single outstanding factor to which a probable causal

---

* Bloodstein, O., *A Handbook on Stuttering*, (Chicago National Easter Seal Society for Crippled Children and Adults, 1969)

** I have replaced the word 'stutter' with 'stammer'

relationship has been most clearly established is competitive pressure for achievement or conformity.

There is a high familial incidence of stammering, and some form of genetic contribution appears to be a distinct possibility.

No major differences between stammerers and non-stammerers in constitution or personality have been discovered, but mild degrees of maladjustment seem to be fairly common, and there may be differences in certain subtle innate or acquired response tendencies.

Stammerers are often somewhat delayed in speech and language development and often tend to have difficulties of articulation.

A fairly large proportion of parents of stammerers appear to be, in varying degrees, demanding, overanxious or perfectionistic in their child-training practices.

Finally, of several major current concepts, the one that seems to be favoured at the moment by the weight of evidence is that stammering is an anticipatory reaction of struggle or avoidance.

Most of these conclusions seem to fit together fairly well. They appear to lend themselves to the inference that stammering usually develops in essentially normal children, at least in part because of certain environmental pressures that induce them to struggle with their attempts at speech and to the view that both hereditary factors and acquired personality traits of certain kinds may play a part in some way.'

A fictional case history

NEWCASTLE UPON TYNE DISTRICT HEALTH AUTHORITY

SPEECH THERAPY UNIT

Name: Benjamin Brown

Address: 1 Any Place
Tynestone
Newcastle upon Tyne

Tel. No.: 123123

Date of birth: 5.1.83

Age/sex: 4.00 years/ M

School: (due April '87)

Code: M = mother
F = father
B = Benjamin

Record No.: 1001

Referee: Family doctor

First attended: 2.2.87

Family doctor: Dr Smith

Address: The Health Centre
Tynestone
Newcastle upon Tyne

Speech therapist: A.I.

Diagnosis: Stammer

Discharged: 22.8.88

Case history from M and F – both came + Ben

Family: Father, mother, John aged 6, Ben just 4.
Four live together, no one else lives with them.
No particular family problems – except stammer.
B and John get on well together, a few brotherly
squabbles, e.g., B taking John's toys, not often.

Family history of stammer: F's brother had quite severe
stammer as a child. Still stammers slightly. They rarely meet
as brother lives in South. No other history known.

Development: Normal pregnancy. Full-term. Normal delivery.
Weaning OK. Sat five months; walked alone twelve months.
M cannot remember details but everything was normal. No

problems recalled, apart from crying when teething.
Illnesses: Ear infection at 12 months; chicken pox two years.

Speech development: Babbled normally. First words at about 12 months (dada and byebye); other details forgotten but phrases well before two and sentences by two and a half years. Mispronounced some words, e.g., car = tar. Was not always intelligible to people outside the family. It didn't present a problem as family always understood him. Pronunciation now OK. M says he's a chatterbox at home; a bit reserved with visitors.

Stammer: Began at about three and a half years, no cause known. Had been talking in sentences without stammer for about one year. It came on gradually – tended to come and go – then got more persistent and M went to GP. He said B would grow out of it. M and F worried as it didn't improve. After 2 months went back to GP who referred him here.

Parents cannot describe stammer – except that it occurs at the beginning of words and mostly at beginning of sentences. Both very worried about it – M particularly anxious, 'Especially when it is bad and it can get very bad, it's been awful during the last few weeks.' Stammer most noticeable when B excited, they think, but occurs at any time. May go an hour or two without stammer – not longer – but it varies from day to day. They tell him to 'slow down' or 'stop and start again' and this usually stops the stammer – many times daily. Granny (maternal) also tells him to 'slow down' and to 'stop getting excited.' John has never mentioned stammer and parents have never mentioned it to him. B has never shown any concern over stammer until, recently, he has twice said 'I can't say it.'

With Ben: Talked with him while we played with toys (parents in room). Outgoing, friendly, chatty. Stammer = repeats sounds (I I I I want, w w w when) and syllables (do do do you, John John John.) Mostly at beginning of sentences, some mid-sentence. Seemed unaware of stammer: M said about it, 'That's it – that's what I mean.' Clearly tension in stammers but not severe. Some gentle repetitions with no apparent tension, sounded like excessive normal non-fluencies.

Parents corrected him (matter of fact, not cross) for very minor offences – twisting the strap of his sandal, banging two cars together – 'Don't do that.' Too high standards?

School: Not yet. Has not been to play group. Home with M. Starts nursery (reception class of infants school) after Easter and school proper next September. (I'll ring nursery teacher at beginning of term to make sure no one reacts negatively to the stammer and ask teachers not to ask a lot of questions.) M worried about his starting nursery in case he gets teased re. speech. Reassured her that children of that age don't tease about speech, don't notice it.

Action: See parents weekly as long as necessary (not see B). M can come weekly; F will come when free – can sometimes manage flexitime. Friends will look after children so that parents can attend. Teach Preventive Therapy. M and F anxious to know if B will get over stammer. Told them it is almost certain that he will if they carry out the Preventive Therapy, although they may find some parts difficult to accept and hard work to carry out. Keen to know what to do, explained we can only take one step at a time.

Just start on Umbrella therapy today so that they have something to work on. Explain that they need to stop reacting negatively to the stammer – in every way. Begin to behave as if B's speech is normal. NO correction of stammer – may correct automatically to start with, but learn to stop correcting it. Explain most important thing is for B to enjoy speaking and not to learn to worry about it. Correcting will make him worry about his speech – worrying about stammering is far more harmful to him than stammering.

No time for detail today but given a notebook (to bring each time) and asked to list what they think makes the stammer (1) increase and (2) decrease so they get guidelines of what situations to try to promote and what to try to avoid. Appointment one week from now – both M and F can come. (M told B to 'say thank you' as they left.)

9/2

M and F came.

When they got home last week and talked about our meeting they could not believe it is right to stop telling B to slow down – 'it is the one thing that stops him stammering.' They did stop correcting him but don't feel happy about it – and say his stammer is just the same!

Plenty of time today: discussed Umbrella therapy in detail and now they really do understand the danger of correction and seem happy to go ahead with it. (I'd told them to regard the stammer as *my* responsibility; I'm confident about the outcome – but only if they carry out the therapy.)

We listed everyone else who talks with B. Neighbours, (maternal) granny and grandpa, B's friends (mostly neighbours' children), M's friends, parents' friends, i.e., 'couples', relations.

M will tell all of them (not B's friends and not John) not to take any notice of the stammer whatsoever and not to 'help' by telling him to take his time, etc. If any disagreements (e.g., granny) can say 'that's what the speech therapist has asked.' Make sure that *nobody* reacts to stammer. (Use notebook to write down anything they wish to discuss so nothing gets forgotten.)

Discussed any other negative reactions to the stammer, including their body language. Told them they both looked anxious last week when B stammered and that M reacted anxiously when she said, 'That's it – that's what I mean.'

I also mentioned them saying 'Don't do that' for trivial offences – are their standards rather unnecessarily high? Discussed. They didn't think so – then said, 'Well, perhaps a bit.'

Notebook: Stammer increased
  ● when excited
  ● talking quickly
  ● couldn't get own way
  ● M's friend in for tea
  ● When all family together

Stammer decreased
  ● when alone at home with M

So
(1) play down excitement
(2) make sure B has *plenty of time* to talk (he may feel pressed when all family at home.)

M and F will continue increase/decrease list. Also notice if their standards are unnecessarily high. Note if they react to stammer with body language (will observe each other for this.)

Told parents that, when stammer begins to improve, it will not be continuous progress, that there are always setbacks. Not to get worried when this happens, it always happens, but soon picks up again. See one week.

16/2

M came alone this week; F working.

M has told 'all in environment' not to take any notice of stammer. Granny disagreed at first but M explained why it was necessary, then she understood and agreed. Parents not feeling so anxious about stammer. M thinks it is as frequent as before but with less tension. B has not said, 'I can't say it' any more.

Discussed again high standards in the home – M and F have noticed some and cut down. Suggest they cut out saying 'don't do that' unless it is necessary as it will cause B frustrations – try to avoid frustrations. M agrees – hadn't really noticed until recently that they were doing it.

M feels that they have the Umbrella therapy under control now, so started on Question therapy today. Explained in detail, examples given of saying as much as usual, but not in question form. M says they (and especially she) ask a lot of questions. They like to show an interest in all of B's activities. Said she had never thought that asking questions could increase the stammer – had thought the opposite, that showing an interest would help him (I explained that showing an interest is good – and also possible without questions!) She understood but thinks it will be hard to do. Will explain everything to F.

From 9/2: M and F have noticed each other reacting to stammer with body language, when B stammering more than usual, e.g., M sighed with relief when B finished telling a story; F looked expectant while waiting. (Parents putting a lot of thought into the therapy.)

They've noticed that B definitely stammers more when he talks quickly and this happens mostly when he is excited. They are trying to play down excitement and make sure he is not excited before bedtime, but say he is rather excitable by nature. Also working on never hurrying his speech and trying not to hurry him over anything.

23/2

M and F. today.

They are delighted! Say they can see a definite change in B's stammer. Less severe and less frequent. They say it is since they began really cutting down the number of questions. Both finding it hard to replace questions with non-question speech (and practise together in the evenings when the children are in bed! They're great!) Practised here. They say they need at least another week to get this under control, so we went over everything we have done so far. Everything sounds fine. Nobody is correcting, body language minimal, working on avoiding time pressure and he's beginning to improve. Good start. See in a week.

2/3

M came.

They are getting on well with Question therapy but feel they need another week on it. They have cut down to only a few questions daily but sometimes still have difficulty in replacing a question with a non-question. So, relaxed session with no further therapy. Did three things (plus coffee!)

(1)   M gave examples of questions she may want to ask B and I suggested ways of putting them into non-question form.

(2)   Discussed, once more, the 'highish standards.' We tried to sort out what seem necessary standards as against what could be called nagging.

(3)   M talked about B starting nursery (27th April), still a bit worried about B's stammer at school. Told her I'd ring teacher. (He has been to see the school, and is looking forward to it.) M will also have a word with teacher and say they are coming for therapy, that B's stammer is improving and not to take any notice of it.

Re. increase/decrease stammer. M has noticed that stammer increases if someone fails to understand what B says and he has to repeat it. Suggest they make a guess at what he said rather than ask him to repeat. Failing this, try, 'Sorry, I wasn't listening properly' instead of, 'What did you say?' and see what happens – let me know.

9/3

M came.

Question therapy going well – 'it seems to be coming naturally now.' M and F have noticed further stammer change in that B is sometimes going longer without stammering. He has been full half days without stammer instead of an hour or two. Now that they are not telling him to slow down they notice the stammer less. They are not sure how much is 'less stammer' and how much is them not feeling the need to notice it and correct it.

Further improvement: B seems more confident with M's best friend who often visits. He talks with her much more than he used to. The friend tends to ask B a lot of questions, so M explained about cutting out questions if possible.

Did Demanding Speech therapy today. M thinks this will be easy after the Question therapy! She doesn't think they demand speech a lot, but will be on the lookout from now on. I told M that on our first meeting she had told B to 'say thank you' as they left. Agrees that she often says 'say thank you' and 'say goodbye.' I suggested that, when B starts nursery, she will need to remember not to keep asking B to tell his father what he has been doing at school.

I'm away next week. See in 2 weeks – 23rd.

23/3

M and F.

They are feeling much less anxious about B now that they are sure the stammer is improving. Then said, 'We'll never feel really sure until it has gone altogether', but they feel 'much more hopeful now.'

The Demanding Speech therapy was comparatively easy – they demanded speech a few times but soon got used to not telling him what to say. They catch themselves on the point of demanding, then usually manage to avoid it. They have found it helpful to remember that anything they say to B that begins with 'say' or 'tell' is to be avoided.

All well – so go on to Interrupting therapy. Both ways, i.e., them not to interrupt B but allow him to interrupt them.

They were not too happy about this. They are happy not to
interrupt him, but thinks B interrupting them is bad for discipline. I explained that we could discuss general discipline
another time but that, in overcoming stammering, there is to
be no speech discipline. It has to be postponed till B is OK. I
said my expectations of the stammer being overcome were
greatly reduced if they insisted on discipline for B's speech.
Other discipline yes, but not speech discipline. Asked them
to think it over, try it out and let me know how they feel next
visit. See one week.

30/3

M and F.

Setback, both 'worried sick'. B was bitten by a dog, took
him to Dr. It wasn't serious but he got quite a shock and his
stammer went right back to how it was before they came.
Reassured them it is sure to pick up again, maybe 2/3 weeks.
Try not to listen to every stammer but, instead, concentrate
carefully on what B says to divert their attention from the
stammer. They wanted to bring him today to 'show me how
bad he is.' If they really want to bring him then bring him next
week, but me hearing him will not help – I'm certain he'll pick
up again. If he comes it will just be a play session so that his
speech is not mentioned (he still seems unaware of stammer.)
Leave it open for them to decide what to do next week.

They haven't done much about Interruption therapy as
they have been preoccupied with the dog episode and
relapse so we discussed in more detail what we had discussed
on last visit. They have already decided to let Benjamin
interrupt them – that's good. They have worked very hard
and need a break – especially as so worried at the moment.
Suggest they take the week off from additional therapy or
could just begin on Interruption therapy if they want to.

6/4

M and F (without B!)

B's stammer has lessened quite a lot already – M and F
relieved. M said her main worry had been that B is almost
due to start nursery school and she didn't want him to start
while his stammer was so bad. Is feeling much happier now
that he has improved so quickly. They have started on the

Interruption therapy – find it hard to remember but feel they have made a good start. Discussed' details of therapy problems that have arisen during the week.

M mentioned that B seems to be going through a 'naughty phase' – has had two temper tantrums and says 'no' when M asks him to do things, e.g., put toys away. Suggest that they go easy with him – he may be reacting to recent events. Discussed general discipline: they have rules but not a lot and they all sound sensible. They occasionally give in after saying 'no', but not often. No real problems with discipline till last week. See what happens and discuss again. (M and F think they have stopped saying 'don't do that' regarding unimportant matters – see 16/2.)

13/4

M came.

Joy! B's stammer is almost back to how it was before the dog bite. No more temper tantrums – and she has tried not to ask him to do things to avoid him refusing to do it.

Parents doing well with not interrupting/allowing interruptions. They are very conscientious – M says they are glad to have plenty to work on! Told her we haven't much more to do now.

Today did Giving Attention therapy, in detail. M doesn't think this will be too difficult as they are used to listening to what he says. Says John usually listens too – and never seems to notice the stammer. She will tell F about what we did today.

I warned M that stammer may increase when B starts nursery. See in two weeks – bank holiday next week.

27/4

M came.

B started nursery today – M a bit anxious for him.

Attention therapy has not presented problems. They've noticed themselves more since being aware of needing to listen when B speaks and still think that they do this automatically.

Says they have hardly noticed B stammering this week – goes a full day without stammering and the stammers now seem to be mostly gentle repetitions of sounds. This is excellent. We agreed that it will be fine to go on to fortnightly sessions now.

Therapy today – Competing for the Chance to Speak. M says it happens occasionally with John and she manages by saying 'one at a time.' See in two weeks.

I rang nursery teacher, told her B had stammer, that now much improved, not to react to it, etc. She had not noticed stammer today but agreed to treat it as normal speech if it occurs.

11/5

M came.

B is loving nursery and it does not affect his stammer. That is great news – it looks as if the stammer is well on the way out for it not to be affected by beginning school. Tell M this.

Therapy today – Pronunciation and Grammar. They don't correct pronunciation as it's OK. Both F and M occasionally correct his grammar ('it's not me and John, it's John and I') – they will stop doing this.

M relieved B happy at school and enjoys a bit more time to herself. Just chatted today. Family going to Yugoslavia for summer hols. See three weeks due to bank holiday.

1/6

Failed to attend. (M rang later – she had asked F to come and he forgot. Good sign – less anxious!) See next week.

8/6

F came (M not too fit).

B still goes a full day without stammer, sometimes longer. Just repeats sounds at the beginning of a sentence – no longer noticed to repeat syllables. Repetitions are still quite easy – very little tension in them.

M and F have noticed that there is rather more competing for chance to speak since nursery started (when John comes in from school both children may speak at the same time, parents tell them to take turns.)

Everything seems to be going very well. To keep all the Preventive Therapy going and write down any problems in the notebook. So, to try coming monthly. Appointment given for July 6, but to ring me if the stammer increases.

6/7

M came.

Stammer continues to improve. Now goes two or three days without stammer. Still occurs when B gets excited – it increased when he had been to a party but settled down in two days. Parents not unduly anxious as they realized what had caused the stammer to increase.

They go to Yugoslavia in about three weeks so I'll not see them for five weeks. Quite a long break until next appointment so we went over the six direct speech pressures.

M says discipline problems are minor, don't present a problem, and M and F have lowered their previous rather high standards for him and make a point of not putting any unnecessary pressures on B.

I think the end of therapy is in sight now – parents are delighted with B's progress.

Reminded M to try to avoid over-excitement about the hols. See Aug 10 (two days after they get back.)

10/8

M and F.

B started stammering 'as soon as he got on the plane'!! His stammer was 'terrible all the time we were there.' They were 'devastated.' They think he was excited by going on a plane for the first time, then many people only spoke Yugoslavian (e.g., waiters) and B seemed very confused and quite frightened. Parents then realized B didn't know that English is not the only language. He couldn't sleep, was bad tempered, cried easily.

Spent session trying to reassure them that the stammer *will* reduce again. I've warned them about setbacks, they agree, but didn't think the stammer 'could get so bad again once it had nearly gone.' See next week.

17/8

M came.

Stammer beginning to get much better. Relief all round! 'Nothing like as good as it has been' but 'definitely much better' and parents are regaining confidence. Discuss the need to be extra careful not to subject B to any pressures and to try to keep the household calm. See three weeks as bank hol. To ring me if any relapse.

7/9

M came.

B started 'big school' today. Quite happy about it. M to speak to new teacher about the stammer and I will ring her.

Everything is fine! B back to how he was before Yugoslavia. Reminded M that path to fluency is never straight – often two steps forward and one back. I think parents realize that now, although M said 'Do you think it will ever go?' Answer, 'Yes, there has been a tremendous improvement in the seven months.' Suggest it is better to be patient – instead of hoping for a particular date when they can declare the stammer gone. Suggest they try – again – not to listen for stammers and count them – but listen to what B *says*.

My hol. now so see them in one month.

5/10

M came.

B very happy at school. Stammer has 'picked up tremendously' – that's good news. He can go at least a week with no stammer and parents not sure if he is actually stammering now as he just repeats sounds gently (at beginning of occasional sentences), but some days are definitely more non-fluent than others, so it looks as if stammer nearly gone but with a little remaining on some days.

See in two months. Ring me if any worries.

30/11

M came.

Everything fine. Parents have not noticed stammer at all during the last few weeks. They are over the moon. Told M – please *don't* be over the moon. The signs are very good but we are not yet home and dry. B could still get setbacks. Let's just relax and see what happens.

Try not to let B get too excited over Christmas – aim to

have fun when Christmas comes but avoid weeks of excitement.

Told M that I'd like to see her in three months (but contact me meantime if problems).

Remind M that when B overcomes his stammer he will still be normally non-fluent, like we all are.

(I'm delaying reintroducing the speech pressures in view of his setbacks + the excitement of Christmas soon.)

22/2

M came.

No stammer over the three months. Told M that I'd like to see her and Benjamin in about six months' time, as a final check. Unlikely to stammer again but it is certainly not out of the question.

Meantime, parents to gradually reintroduce the six speech pressures – all explained to M in detail, so that B will again be treated as every other child, with pressures on speech, but to do it gradually and to stop any pressure if it causes stammering.

22/8

M came with B.

Happy day. B is fine.

All speech pressures have been reintroduced.

No stammer in last nine months.

Discharged.

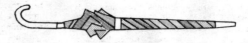

Index